WITHDRAWN FROM
BROMLEY LIBRARIES

To renew, find us online at:

https://capitadiscovery.co.uk/bromley

Please note: Items from the adult library
may also accrue overdue charges when
borrowed on children's tickets.

In partnership with

ORPINGTON LIBRARY
01689 831551

BETTER
the feel good place

PENGUIN LIFE EXPERTS SERIES

The Penguin Life Experts series equips readers with simple but vital information on common health issues and empowers readers to get to know their own bodies to better improve their health. Books in the series include:

Managing Your Migraine
by Dr Katy Munro

* * * * *

Preparing for the Perimenopause and Menopause
by Dr Louise Newson

* * * * *

Next in the series, publishing in 2021 and 2022:

Keeping Your Heart Healthy
by Dr Boon Lim

* * * * *

Understanding Allergy
by Dr Sophie Farooque

* * * * *

Managing IBS
by Dr Lisa Das

Preparing for the Perimenopause and Menopause

DR LOUISE NEWSON

PENGUIN LIFE

AN IMPRINT OF

PENGUIN BOOKS

PENGUIN LIFE

UK | USA | Canada | Ireland | Australia
India | New Zealand | South Africa

Penguin Life is part of the Penguin Random House group of companies
whose addresses can be found at global.penguinrandomhouse.com.

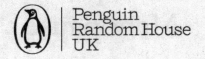

First published 2021

004

Copyright © Dr Louise Newson, 2021

The moral right of the author has been asserted

Set in 12.5/14.75 pt Garamond MT Std
Typeset by Jouve (UK), Milton Keynes
Printed and bound in Great Britain by Clays Ltd, Elcograf S.p.A.

The authorized representative in the EEA is Penguin Random House Ireland,
Morrison Chambers, 32 Nassau Street, Dublin D02 YH68

A CIP catalogue record for this book is available from the British Library

ISBN: 978–0–241–50464–2

www.greenpenguin.co.uk

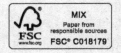

MIX
Paper from
responsible sources
FSC® C018179

Penguin Random House is committed to a
sustainable future for our business, our readers
and our planet. This book is made from Forest
Stewardship Council® certified paper.

To my family, who constantly listen to my ideas, plans and also frustrations about my work and give me the encouragement and support to work so hard.

Contents

Introduction: What the Menopause Is and Why It Happens

I was in my mid-forties when it started. By day, I felt hot, bothered and weighed down by crushing fatigue. Night after night I would wake up drenched in sweat. I was short-tempered and irritable with my husband and three daughters. Poor concentration levels meant I was terrified of making a mistake in my busy job as a GP.

A throwaway comment from my eleven-year-old daughter, suggesting that I was short-tempered because my period was due, made me recall that I hadn't actually had a period for many months. I realized that it wasn't pre-menstrual syndrome I was suffering from: I was peri-menopausal.

It sounds strange that, as a menopause specialist, I couldn't recognize what my body was telling me. Yet my experience underscores that we often fail to realize what huge life events the perimenopause and menopause are for women.

Doctors frequently misdiagnose them, and society shies away from talking about menopause, filing it away under 'women's problems'. But the menopause is something almost every woman will go through – and it can happen sooner than you think. An estimated one in twenty women will go through the menopause between the ages of forty and forty-five, and one in 100 before the age of forty. And research has shown that more than one-third of perimeno-pausal and menopausal women in the UK wait at least a year to receive adequate treatment for their symptoms; and for one in ten women, it takes more than nine doctor's appointments even to make the diagnosis.

There should be no stigma or shame attached to the menopause. Not openly discussing it can add up to a potential physical and mental-health time-bomb for women, both now and in later life. We need to stop label-ling the menopause as a natural process when women resign themselves to years of misery and simply have no choice but to endure the symptoms.

Instead we should be calling it what it actually is: a long-term hormone deficiency, which, with the right support, treatments and lifestyle changes, can be managed so that the symptoms improve and, more importantly, women's future health improves. We need to start de-stigmatizing the menopause, so that all women have a better under-standing of it and greater control of their own bodies.

After my own perimenopause diagnosis I set up www.menopausedoctor.co.uk, my website that provides unbiased and evidence-based information about the perimenopause and menopause. I then decided to open my own practice specializing in menopause care, called Newson Health. Since we opened our doors in 2018 we have helped thousands of people to receive individual-ized advice and support to tackle their perimenopause and menopause. Frustratingly, I was unable to open an NHS menopause clinic as there was insufficient funding and interest for this.

De-stigmatizing menopause was what also motivated me to set up the Menopause Charity in 2020 (www.themenopausecharity.org), dedicated to raising awareness of, and removing embarrassment around, the perimenopause and menopause. Part of the charity's mission is to develop a helpline to really assist women. In 2020 I also launched my free Balance app (balance-app.com), which has been designed to empower women. I'm passionate that women can talk openly about their experiences and have access to clear, unbiased information and support so they can take charge of their own health and well-being.

Maybe you are in the middle of the menopause and are looking for advice on how to tackle troublesome symptoms, or perhaps you haven't had any symptoms yet and want to prepare yourself for the perimenopause. It is never too late – or too early – to be perimenopause- and menopause-savvy.

Over the course of this book I'll take you through everything you need to know in order to prepare and get through the perimenopause and menopause: the causes, the symptoms and, importantly, the treatments and life-style advice that can make this stage of your life as healthy, stress-free and symptom-free as possible. After reading this book you will feel empowered to embrace 'the change', take charge of your health and ensure that you receive the best possible treatment, which is individualized for you.

Along the way you will also hear from women of all ages and backgrounds on how they overcame their perimenopause- and menopause-related challenges, to remind you that you certainly aren't alone.

What are the perimenopause and menopause?

Your menopause is when you stop having periods. It occurs when your ovaries stop producing eggs and, as a result, levels of hormones called oestrogen and progesterone fall. You can split the process into four stages:

- **Pre-menopause**: The time in your life before any menopausal symptoms occur
- **Perimenopause**: When you experience menopausal symptoms due to hormone changes but still have your periods, which are changing in nature or frequency
- **Menopause**: When you do not have a period for twelve consecutive months
- **Post-menopause**: The time in your life after you have not had a period for twelve consecutive months.

When do the perimenopause and menopause happen?

A bit like when you start having periods, every woman's experience is different. What we do know is that the average age of the menopause is fifty-one, so most women can expect to start having symptoms of the perimenopause at around forty-five years of age. These symptoms can start to occur even a decade before your periods finally stop.

If the menopause happens when a woman is under forty-five, we call it an **early menopause**. If it occurs before the age of forty, it is classed as **Premature ovarian insufficiency** (POI). Many women in their twenties, thirties and forties will be perimenopausal without even realizing it, and some will not even know what the perimenopause actually is.

Will my menopause mainly consist of hot flushes and my periods stopping?

Yes and no.

The hormones oestrogen and progesterone work together to regulate the menstrual cycle and the production of eggs. Your ovaries also produce the hormone testosterone. But it's not simply about your reproductive system. We have oestrogen receptors in every cell throughout our bodies. Name a function in your body and the chances are that oestrogen will play an important part in keeping things running smoothly: oestrogen plays a key role in everything from our memory, mood, immune function and heart, to our muscles and even our hair and skin.

During your perimenopause and menopause, hormone levels fluctuate greatly, leaving you with a hormone deficiency. I tend to liken it to a car running on empty. And it is this hormone deficiency that can trigger a range of symptoms, from the hot flushes that everyone associates with the menopause, through to joint pains, mood changes and even memory lapses. We will cover the full range of symptoms in the coming chapters.

> <u>Tip</u>: **Talk to female members of your family –
> your mother, grandmother, sisters – about
> when they went through their menopause. We
> sometimes find that women whose mother or
> grandmother had an earlier or later menopause
> may follow suit.**

Do I need to get a menopause diagnosis?

In the vast majority of cases there is no one definitive test
to diagnose the menopause. Instead it is about looking at
your age and the type of symptoms you are having.

Irregular periods can be an early first sign. If you are over
forty-five, have irregular periods and other typical perimenopausal and menopausal symptoms, then a healthcare
professional should be able to diagnose your menopause
without the need for tests.

Sadly, however, a large number of healthcare professionals have not had the menopause training needed to
recognize the range of symptoms, meaning that some
women may go through months, or even years, of mis-
diagnosis. This means they are often suffering needlessly
from their symptoms, and their future health may be at risk
without the right help, support and treatment.

This is why it is essential that we are tuned into our
bodies, so that we can keep track of any changes in our
physical and mental health – and this book will help you on
your journey. By empowering you with the knowledge to
understand the perimenopause and menopause, the ability

to recognize the signs and symptoms, and the right tools to enable you to speak to your healthcare professional with confidence, you should be able to ask the right questions and secure yourself the best possible treatment.

1. Change before 'The Change': the Perimenopause

The perimenopause will probably begin with a small, barely noticeable change to your periods. Perhaps they come a little earlier or even a little later than you would usually expect. They may be lighter and shorter one month and heavier the next. Things may settle down for a while, but a few months down the line you may find it increasingly hard to concentrate at work, and feel irritable at home. You might generally feel that life is a bit more of a struggle than it used to be.

You bump into an old school friend and feel embarrassed when you can't recall their name. You put it down to a lack of sleep – after all, it's been weeks since you managed a night without waking up at least once, hasn't it? Maybe you don't make the instant connection between all these events, but one thing is for sure: you don't feel quite like 'you'.

What I have described here is a fairly typical experience of the perimenopause, the stage directly before the menopause. But with so much emphasis on the menopause itself, you could be forgiven for not realizing quite how disruptive the perimenopause can actually be. With very few exceptions (such as surgery to remove the ovaries), the menopause is the culmination of a gradual process and not a short, sharp event. The perimenopause is the start of the process and can actually last for many months or years.

In this chapter we look at the science behind the peri-menopause: *why* it happens and *how* it happens, so that you are better informed about what to expect.

All about hormones

Oestrogen and progesterone are the driving forces behind our menstrual cycle, the monthly hormonal process whereby a woman's body prepares for possible pregnancy. Oestrogen levels in our bodies are largely controlled by

Fallopian tubes – connect the ovaries to the uterus

Uterus (womb) – where a fertilized egg and baby develop

Ovaries – where eggs develop and are released

Myometrium (lining of the womb) – this lining sheds to lead to bleeding and periods

Cervix – entrance to the uterus from the vagina

Vagina

Female reproductive system

hormones known as follicle-stimulating hormone (FSH) and luteinizing hormone (LH).

FSH stimulates our ovaries to produce oestrogen, and when oestrogen reaches a certain level, the pituitary gland in our brains switches off the FSH and produces a surge of LH. This triggers the ovary to release an egg (known as ovulation). The ovary then produces progesterone and oestrogen to prepare the uterus for possible pregnancy. As levels of these hormones rise, so the levels of FSH and LH drop. If the egg isn't fertilized, then progesterone falls, menstruation happens and the cycle starts again.

What hormonal changes happen during the perimenopause?

For most women, our oestrogen and progesterone levels rise and fall pretty consistently in line with our

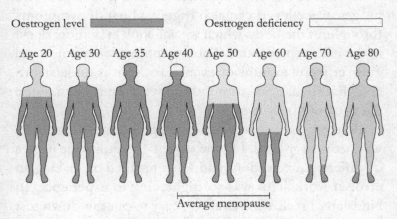

Oestrogen level | Oestrogen deficiency

Age 20　Age 30　Age 35　Age 40　Age 50　Age 60　Age 70　Age 80

Average menopause

Women's oestrogen levels by decade

menstrual cycle. But as we approach the menopause, our ovaries make fewer and fewer of these hormones and our fertility starts to decline until we reach a point, after our menopause, where we are no longer able to get pregnant.

The perimenopause signals the start of this process and is a time when our hormones are in a state of flux.

How can I tell if I am perimenopausal?

Typically the first sign may be changes to the frequency, duration or flow of your periods. But it isn't always easy to make the connection. Because hormone levels are fluctuating, many women will have a completely normal period one month, then it can be heavier or is missed altogether, before going back to normal again for a few months.

The knock-on effect of these fluctuating oestrogen and progesterone levels can also trigger a host of symptoms throughout the body, which we will look at in more detail in the next two chapters. These symptoms may come and go over many months or even years, so it is understandable that so many of us put these symptoms down to the stress of our busy lives.

Take my experience, for example: before I realized I was perimenopausal, I found myself forgetting the names of different medications and I was terrified of making an error at work. This was so frightening to experience. In hindsight, I realize it was all too easy to put this down to a busy work and home life.

When will the perimenopause start and do I need a diagnosis?

Like the menopause, there is no set age at which the peri-menopause will start, but for most women it is likely to be around forty-five years of age. For many women it is much younger, though.

If you suspect you might be perimenopausal, see a healthcare professional. As with the menopause, if you are forty-five or older a healthcare professional should be able to make a diagnosis on account of changes to your periods and any other symptoms that you may be experiencing. You do not need a hormone blood test (which will be unreliable anyway).

Read through the rundown of perimenopause and menopause symptoms in the next two chapters and note down any that you are experiencing. Keeping a record of your symptoms, and how they change over time, can help aid a diagnosis. A really useful tool to do this is the menopause symptom sheet on my website (tinyurl.com/menopausedoctor-symptom-sheet), which is reproduced below.

Symptom	Not at all 0	A little 1	Quite often 2	Extremely often 3	Comment
Heart beating quickly or strongly					
Feeling tense/ nervous					

Symptom	Not at all 0	A little 1	Quite often 2	Extremely often 3	Comment
Trouble sleeping					
Feeling excitable					
Panic or anxiety attacks					
Difficulty concentrating					
Tiredness or lack of energy					
Loss of interest in most things					
Feeling unhappy					
Crying spells					
Feeling irritable					
Feeling faint or dizzy					
Pressure or tightness in the head					
Headaches					
Numbness in parts of the body					
Muscle and/or joint pains					

Symptom	Not at all 0	A little 1	Quite often 2	Extremely often 3	Comment
Loss of feeling in the hands or feet					
Breathing difficulties					
Hot flushes					
Night sweats					
Loss of interest in sex					

Symptom sheet

You could also use my free Balance app (balance-app. com), which has been downloaded by thousands of women in more than 100 countries. It contains advice and enables you to record your symptoms, moods, periods, nutrition, exercise and meditation. It contains a huge amount of information, and there is the ability to download a Health Report for you to take to your healthcare professional too.

What treatment might help?

Rest assured, there are a lot of effective treatments available. Many symptoms of the perimenopause and menopause overlap, so this means that you will usually benefit from the same advice and treatments offered during the menopause. We will be covering the range of treatments that can help later in the book (see Chapter 4), including hormone replacement therapy (HRT).

There is a common misconception that you can only start treatment once you are actually in the menopause. This isn't true: if your symptoms are affecting your day-to-day life, don't wait. The earlier a woman receives treatment, the more benefits to her future health there will be. Speak to a healthcare professional about possible treatments in order to make an informed decision.

How will I know when I have moved from perimenopause to the menopause?

While many perimenopausal and menopausal symptoms overlap, the key difference is this: while in the perimeno-pause, your periods may change in frequency, flow or duration; the menopause is when you do not have a period for twelve consecutive months.

Claire, 42

Claire had always been fit, healthy and a 'glass half-full' kind of woman, but on turning forty, everything changed. For the first time in her life she began suffering unbearable migraines and heart palpitations. She had terrible anxiety that came from nowhere, was irritable with her husband and two children and felt zapped of energy. Even the most mundane tasks, such as unloading the washing machine, became a challenge, due to brain fog.

Three months after turning forty, Claire had the first of many GP appointments to try and get to the bottom of why she was feeling this way. She would turn up with a long list of ailments at each visit, and her doctor prescribed sumatriptan for her migraines, but the medication made her feel sick and groggy. After sobbing at yet another appointment, Claire was prescribed citalopram, an anti-anxiety medication, which she hoped would be the answer; but she stopped taking it after six months because it didn't make any difference.

Claire was desperate to try anything. She was given an echocardiogram for the palpitations, but it showed that her heart was perfectly normal. Looking back, Claire says she now realizes it was around this time that her periods changed, with some months being lighter and shorter than others. But neither Claire nor her doctor made the link that she could be heading towards the menopause.

At another appointment Claire was handed a prescription for beta-blockers, which slow the heart rate and can help with anxiety, but they left her feeling spaced out and sluggish.

It was during a routine asthma check-up for her son at the same surgery that the penny dropped, when she overheard a lady in the waiting room talking about her menopause. Tearfully, Claire told a friendly nurse about her symptoms.

'You're not going crazy – you're perimenopausal,' the nurse said, explaining how her symptoms were probably due to changing hormone levels.

At first Claire dismissed the idea as she was only forty-one, surely too young to be perimenopausal. She was prescribed the progestogen-only pill, but although this helped with the migraines and the anxiety, it caused heavy bleeding (the progestogen-only pill is not a treatment for the perimenopause).

It was at this point that Claire came to see me. Looking at her long list of symptoms, I could see that she was perimenopausal and I prescribed HRT. This simply replaced her missing hormones (so it improved her hormone deficiency, which was occurring as a result of her perimenopause).

It has now been almost a year since Claire started taking HRT and she says the difference has been incredible. Her symptoms have subsided, and instead of feeling as if her best years were behind her, she is looking forward to what the future holds.

Spotlight on contraception

The combined pill, the mini pill, the implant, coils, caps and condoms . . . Millions of women in the UK currently use some form of contraception, and many have done so for most of their adult lives.

So how do the perimenopause and menopause affect the contraceptive choices you make? Here's what you need to know.

Will taking contraception delay or hasten the perimenopause or menopause?

No, but some types of contraception can conceal changes to your periods that may often be an early sign of the perimenopause.

I'm perimenopausal: does that mean I can stop taking contraception?

You could be forgiven for thinking that your perimenopause and menopause herald the end of having to use birth-control pills, injections or implants. Our fertility starts to decline from our mid-thirties, but it is important to remember that you can still produce eggs (ovulate) if you are having periods, even if they are irregular.

If you want to avoid an unplanned pregnancy during your perimenopause and menopause, then you will still need contraception. HRT shouldn't generally be used in place of contraception: it contains only low levels of hormones and therefore does not work as a contraceptive. However, some types of HRT can be used as a contraceptive – for example, women who have the Mirena® coil with oestrogen.

Current guidance advises that women under fifty should use contraception for at least two years following their last menstrual period; and for at least one year after their last period if they are over fifty.[1]

Time for a contraception refresher

More of us are choosing to have children later in life – nearly one in four (22.4 per cent) of live births in England and Wales in 2017 was born to a mother aged thirty-five or above.[2] But there are various types of contraception available, if you want to avoid getting pregnant.

- **Barrier methods:** These include male condoms, female condoms, diaphragms and cervical caps. There are no age restrictions on the use of barrier methods. Barrier methods are crucial if you are in a newer relationship, or where there is a risk of a sexually transmitted infection.
- **Sterilization:** This is a permanent method of contraception for people who are sure they never want children or any more children. Sterilization works by stopping the egg and the sperm meeting.[3] In women this is done by cutting, sealing or blocking the Fallopian tubes that carry an egg from the ovary to the uterus. While a vasectomy (male sterilization) is safe and usually quick and easy to perform, female sterilization is associated with more risks. And it does not alter or stop your periods, so you might find a long-acting contraceptive option more suitable, as this provides additional benefits with regard to your periods, as discussed below.

- **Combined oral contraceptive pill**: This contains both oestrogen and progestogen. It is a popular choice in younger women, but usually needs very careful consideration in those over the age of forty. It should be avoided over the age of thirty-five years if you smoke or are overweight. In women who are fit and healthy – such as those without any cardiovascular risk factors or migraines – taking the pill can have considerable benefits in regulating periods and reducing the heaviness of flow. It can also be used in place of HRT to treat meno-pausal symptoms and prevent osteoporosis in women under the age of fifty. However, the hormones it contains are synthetic and actually present more risks than taking HRT.

- **Progestogen-only pill**: Also known as the 'mini pill', this has fewer risks than the oral contraceptive pill and can be taken at any age, for as long as con-traception is required. Periods can become irregular, stop altogether or last longer when taking this type of pill. It can also sometimes help with heavy, painful periods.

- **Contraceptive injection (Depo-Provera and Sayana Press)**: This is a three-monthly injection of a progestogen. It can be a useful treatment for heavy periods, and is a good option for those who might forget to take a daily pill. However, it might be worth looking at a different option if you have additional risk factors for osteoporosis; and you might want to consider switching to a lower-dose method (for example, the progestogen-only pill or implant) if you are over fifty, as it may be associated with lower bone density in women.

- **Contraceptive implant**: This is a small plastic rod inserted under the skin of the upper arm. It releases progestogen and lasts for three years. Bleeding with this implant can be very variable: periods may become irregular, stop altogether or last for longer. However, the implant may help with heavy, painful periods.

- **Contraceptive coil**: There are two types of coil. The IUCD (copper coil) is hormone-free. If it is inserted after the age of forty, it can be left in place until after the menopause. The IUS (Mirena® coil) contains a small amount of a progestogen hormone that is released gradually. It can be a very useful device during the perimenopause as it has three potential uses – as a contraceptive, a treatment for heavy periods (half of women stop having periods while using it) and by providing the progestogen component of HRT. It needs changing every five years.

Can I use HRT and contraception at the same time?

Barrier methods, the progestogen-only pill, the contraceptive injection and implant can all be safely used alongside HRT. Women with a Mirena® coil as part of their HRT do not need additional contraception.

The hormones in the combined pill cause a monthly withdrawal bleed, which can appear the same as a monthly period. If you are using a progestogen-only contraceptive, such as the progestogen-only pill, implant, injection or Mirena® coil, you might not have any periods at all.

How can I tell if I'm perimenopausal or menopausal while taking contraception?

Keep a note of any symptoms, and a blood test to check your FSH level may be helpful to determine how long you need contraception for. Your doctor should be able to perform this. If your FSH level is elevated, you should continue with contraception for two years if you are under fifty, or for one year if you are over fifty years old.

Note that if you are taking the combined contraceptive pill you will need to stop taking it for at least six weeks before this blood test, as the pill can affect the accuracy of the result – but remember to use adequate alternative protection in the meantime. High doses of progestogens in the injection may also affect the test result.

How long do I need to keep taking contraception?

It is widely agreed to be safe for all women to stop contraception at the age of fifty-five. Natural conception after this age is exceptionally rare, even in women who are still having some periods.

2. What to Expect: Common Symptoms You Need to Know About

There is more to the perimenopause and menopause than hot flushes and changing periods.

In addition to oestrogen regulating our menstrual cycle, cells throughout our bodies are teeming with oestrogen receptors and use this hormone to keep our brain and body in good working order. So when our oestrogen levels become depleted, this can trigger a whole host of symptoms. Our bodies can also be affected by changing levels of progesterone, another hormone involved in the menstrual cycle.

And it might surprise you to read that testosterone also comes into play during the perimenopause and menopause. Although you might think of testosterone as an exclusively 'male' hormone, changing levels of it during this time can cause problems with women's mood, our energy levels and our sex drive.

In this chapter I will be taking you through the most common and lesser-known symptoms of the perimenopause and menopause, explaining how they might make you feel and why they happen.

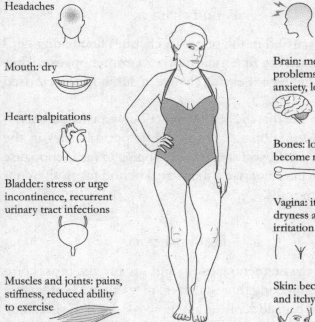

Headaches

Mouth: dry

Heart: palpitations

Bladder: stress or urge
incontinence, recurrent
urinary tract infections

Muscles and joints: pains,
stiffness, reduced ability
to exercise

Hot flushes

Brain: memory
problems, brain fog,
anxiety, low mood

Bones: lose mass and
become more fragile

Vagina: itchiness,
dryness and
irritation

Skin: becomes drier
and itchy

Symptoms and changes linked to
the perimenopause and menopause

Symptoms of the perimenopause and menopause

Here we will look in more detail at the reasons behind
some of the more common – and some of the more
surprising – symptoms that you may experience.

Period changes

As we discussed in the previous chapter, fluctuating periods are often the first indication of perimenopause. They might be lighter or heavier, change in duration or be missed entirely.

Remember that the key difference between the perimenopause and menopause is that while periods vary in the perimenopause, you are classed as being in the menopause when you have not had a menstrual period for twelve consecutive months.

Hot flushes

This is a classic menopause symptom and the most common one, affecting three-quarters of women.[1] Hot flushes can come on suddenly at any time of the day, spreading throughout the face, chest and body. They may be accompanied by other symptoms, such as sweating, dizziness or even heart palpitations.

- **Why do they happen?** The exact reason is not known, but some believe it is because falling oestrogen levels affect noradrenaline, another hormone that regulates our body temperature. Oestrogen also directly affects the thermoregulatory areas of our brains.
- **How many hot flushes a day is 'normal'?** As you will discover over the course of this book, there is

very rarely a 'normal', when it comes to the peri-menopause and menopause. Just as we cannot predict when and how long your menopause will last, so the severity of symptoms varies from woman to woman. And symptoms usually change with time. Hot flushes can happen a few times a week or every day. In the most severe cases, they may occur hourly. The duration often varies too. In some women they may last for moments, and for others several minutes.

Night sweats

Similar to hot flushes but always accompanied by sweating, night sweats are a key reason for sleep disturbance among perimenopausal and menopausal women. As with hot flushes, correcting your hormone deficiency should ease the symptoms of night sweats – and you will find other tips on how to get a good night's sleep in Chapter 7.

Fatigue and disturbed sleep

Many women are plagued by poor sleep during their perimenopause and menopause because oestrogen and testosterone are so important for good-quality sleep. Other symptoms, such as night sweats, can disturb sleep and trigger these reactions.

See Chapter 7 (page 109) for a rundown of the causes of sleep disturbance – and how to get some relief.

Low mood, anxiety and mood swings

These are extremely common symptoms and ones that the majority of women who come to my clinic have trouble coping with. Women tell me how one minute they can be feeling perfectly fine, and the next they are in tears or have bouts of uncontrollable rage.

- **Why does this happen?** Fluctuating oestrogen, progesterone and testosterone levels all contribute to symptoms including low mood, feelings of irritability and even extreme anger. These are such common problems – and ones that are often wrongly diagnosed as clinical depression – that I have devoted a whole chapter to the issue of menopause and mental health (see Chapter 6).

'Brain fog'

Many women use this as a collective term for cognitive issues such as memory and concentration lapses. You might find yourself forgetting names, unable to concentrate at work or simply feel 'foggy'. It's a symptom that can really affect people's careers – I've known women who have left their jobs because they are convinced they have dementia, when in actual fact their brain fog is down to their low hormone levels.

- **Why does this occur?** Hormones are essential in keeping important brain functions such as memory and cognition in good working order. When these hormones become depleted or lower in level, it often leads to symptoms affecting our memory. Other symptoms, such as fatigue and poor sleep, can also make brain fog worse.

Joint aches and pains – why you need to be aware of your osteoporosis risk

Women often complain of soreness and stiffness in their joints (where two bones meet). Oestrogen is very important in providing lubrication for your joints and preventing inflammation, so an oestrogen deficiency can cause aches and pains.

Our bones are a living tissue, which constantly changes throughout our lives in order to be as healthy as possible. You have cells in your body that are constantly laying down new bone (osteoblasts) and other cells that are removing old bone (osteoclasts).

Until you are around thirty years of age you normally build more bone than you lose. However, during the menopause your bone breakdown occurs at a faster rate than your bone build-up, resulting in a loss of bone mass.

Around 10 per cent of a woman's bone mass is lost in the first five years of the menopause and this increases your risk of osteoporosis – a condition that weakens our bones and makes them more likely to break. Other risk factors for osteoporosis include a family history of the condition, the use of some medications such as steroids, and having a low body mass index (BMI). BMI is a calculation that uses a person's height and weight to determine if they are a healthy weight; a level under 18.5 is considered low. Other risk factors for osteoporosis include smoking and drinking alcohol regularly.

If you are diagnosed with osteoporosis, your healthcare professional should take you through the treatment options, which may include hormones, bisphosphonates (medication to slow the rate that bone is broken down in your body) or calcium and vitamin D supplements.

Heart palpitations – and a long-term risk of cardiovascular disease

In the short term the perimenopause and menopause can cause palpitations – that is, a sensation that your heart is beating faster than normal. This can sometimes also happen during a hot flush and is often due to fluctuating hormones, but do see a doctor if you are concerned about any such symptoms.

- **Why are women at increased risk of cardiovascular disease?** The cardiovascular system refers to the heart, arteries, blood vessels and the blood. Oestrogen helps to protect our arteries by reducing the build-up of fatty plaques that can cause the arteries to narrow, meaning that blood and oxygen can't reach our vital organs. It also helps to control our cholesterol levels. Low oestrogen during the perimenopause and after the menopause leads to women having an increased risk of developing cardiovascular disease, which can include heart disease, stroke and vascular dementia. Women who go through an early menopause and do not receive treatment with HRT have an even greater risk of cardiovascular disease and osteoporosis, because their oestrogen levels remain lower for longer.

Worsening migraines

Women are three times more likely than men to suffer from migraines:[2] moderate to severe headaches that often affect one side of the head. Common types include: **migraine with aura** – symptoms that act as a red flag just before a migraine appears, including flashing lights, vertigo, dizziness or tingling sensations; **migraine without aura** – the most common type, where the migraine happens without those specific warning signs; **silent migraine** – where an aura or other migraine symptom is experienced, but a headache doesn't develop.

- **Why does it happen?** Changing hormones, particularly a dip in oestrogen levels, have been found to trigger migraines in some women. For younger women this tends to happen a day or two before their period, or during the seven-day break for those taking the combined oral contraceptive pill.

Migraine without aura can be heavily influenced by the drop in oestrogen levels during perimenopause and menopause. It is very common for migraine without aura to become more frequent and severe at this stage and may coincide with your periods becoming heavier and more erratic. In contrast, migraine with aura tends to increase when your body has higher levels of oestrogen, such as during pregnancy or when taking the combined oral contraceptive pill. When you first take HRT, you may find that you have a short-term increase in the severity or frequency of your migraines because your body is getting used to raised levels of oestrogen, but this usually settles down, and migraines commonly improve.

Migraines can also be brought about by other symptoms, such as hot flushes, night sweats, poor sleep and mood swings. Following a natural menopause the frequency of migraine generally reduces as the hormonal triggers for headaches settle with time, though this could take several years.

Changing body shape and weight gain
A combination of hormone changes, fatigue and stress-induced comfort-eating means it is quite common to gain some weight during the

perimenopause and menopause. The way our bodies store fat also changes. In earlier life, fat is usually distributed around the hips and thighs, but this becomes more concentrated around our middle (the so-called 'spare tyre').[3]

This happens because our bodies start to recognize declining ovarian oestrogen levels and look elsewhere for the hormone, in a weak form of oestrogen produced by fat cells. The body tries to create more of this oestrogen by building up fat stores. Many women might find they develop more fat around the middle in response to the body trying to create a reserve of oestrogen in their fat cells.

Menopausal women also respond differently to glucose (sugar) and are at greater risk of becoming resistant to insulin – the hormone that helps your body use glucose for energy. This can raise the risk of Type 2 diabetes, as well as weight gain.

Lower testosterone levels during perimenopause and menopause can also slow our metabolism, making it harder to shift fat. A decline in testosterone can lead to a decrease in muscle mass and lower energy levels, which in turn can reduce your baseline metabolic rate. This means that you burn fewer calories, even if you have exactly the same nutritional intake as before your perimenopause.[4]

Changes to your breasts

You may notice some changes to the size and shape of your breasts and they may feel tender. Lumps in your breasts can be common too around perimenopause and menopause. These are usually nothing to worry about, but do seek advice from a healthcare professional if you are at all worried.

- **Why does this happen?** Falling oestrogen levels start to affect the milk system in our breasts, causing the glandular tissue to become dehydrated and shrink. Breasts will start to lose their rounded shape and may start to sag.

Skin changes

Skin problems are a common and distressing perimenopausal and menopausal symptom. Women often complain that their skin feels tight, dry and looks dull. Fine lines may appear more prominent, and some women see the return of acne from their younger years. But it is not just the skin on our face that can be affected. Many women suffer from unbearably dry or itchy skin all over their bodies. Some women experience a really unpleasant sensation called 'formication' – that of ants crawling on (or just under) their skin.

- **Why does this occur?** Most of the cells in our skin have oestrogen receptors. Oestrogen has four key functions in our skin:

1. Oestrogen stimulates secretions from our sebaceous glands, known as **sebum**, which keeps our skin lubricated and moisturized.
2. It also produces **hyaluronic acid**, a gel-like substance in the derma layer of the skin just below the skin's surface. Hyaluronic acid is a natural hydration agent and retains water, giving the skin fullness and reducing fine lines and dryness.
3. Oestrogen produces **ceramides**, a lipid or oil that binds together the skin's top layer (epidermis) so that it retains water and protects from irritants.
4. Oestrogen also builds **collagen**, a connective protein that gives our skin structure and strength.

When oestrogen levels fall during perimenopause and menopause, levels of collagen and these natural moisturizing agents – sebum, hyaluronic acid and ceramides – all fall too, so it is unsurprising that we can be left with dry, uncomfortable skin. Some women find their skin actually becomes more spotty and oily during the perimenopause and menopause. This can happen when testosterone changes cause an overproduction of sebum, leading to blocked hair follicles and breakouts.

Caring for your skin during perimenopause and menopause

Dr Sajjad Rajpar is a consultant dermatologist who has appeared as a guest on my podcast

(www.menopausedoctor.co.uk/podcasts) and offers the following advice.

- <u>Look after your hands</u>: Gentle body cleansers such as the CeraVe brand are inexpensive and are kind to your skin. Light moisturizing lotions can also be used in place of soap to cleanse your skin and replenish the moisture every time you wash your hands or body.

- <u>Ditch your loofahs in the shower</u>: Avoid scrubbing at dry or itchy skin – you will be stripping greases as you rub and at the same time stimulating the release of histamine in the skin, causing it to itch even more.

- <u>Wear sunscreen</u>: Falling oestrogen levels mean that the number of cells that produce melanin, which protects our skin from the sun, also decreases. Menopausal skin is therefore more prone to sun damage. Wear a high-factor sunscreen, ideally SPF 50.

Hair changes

Some women find that their hair becomes dry, thinner and less glossy during the perimenopause and menopause. Others find they develop more noticeable facial hair around the lip and chin area, which can affect their self-esteem.

- **Why does this happen?** Lack of oestrogen can affect the texture of our hair, leaving it more prone to breakage. And when oestrogen levels decline, androgens (a collective term for male hormones) sometimes become more prominent. This imbalance of hormones can shrink our hair follicles, making our hair finer, and can also be responsible for facial hair.

Hair tips during perimenopause and menopause

Matthew Curtis is a leading hairdresser who offers the following advice.

Many women find that changing their hair products can make a really positive difference to their hair texture and growth. Using a regular scalp treatment can encourage new hair growth, and changing to a soft bristle brush can reduce the amount of tension on your hair. Many women are using hairdryers that are old, which can parch the hair, causing it to lose moisture and become drier. Updating your hairdryer to one with variable heat settings and even a smart-sensor can really work well for many women.

Oestrogen and COVID-19: What you need to know

The COVID-19 pandemic has been one of the most devastating health crises in living memory, impacting on all our lives in so many ways. Early in the pandemic it became clear that, compared to women, men were at greater risk of severe illness and death from COVID-19. Why is this? Well, emerging evidence is firmly pointing to oestrogen, and to the protective effect of this hormone in a woman's body.

How oestrogen helps protect against infection

As well as my medical degree, I hold a degree in immunology and have for many years been fascinated by the role oestrogen plays in helping our bodies fight infection. We now know all about the protective qualities of oestrogen throughout our bodies, including on our mood, our bones and our cardiovascular system.

But there are also oestrogen receptors in all cells that fight infection, known as immune cells. Oestrogen works to improve the number, the genetic programming and the lifespan of all these immune cells. It also controls the production of cytokines – chemicals that are produced by these immune cells in response to infection. This is crucial, as a large build-up of cytokines (known as a 'cytokine storm') can lead to organ and tissue damage. The cytokine storm can be difficult to switch off, once it becomes active.

In the case of COVID, oestrogen can regulate and reduce the production of cytokines, including one called interleukin-6. This in turn lessens the risk of a cytokine storm developing and then reduces tissue damage, particularly to the respiratory system, which is especially vulnerable to damage from COVID infection. This means that these chemicals do not damage healthy cells.

In addition, the immune cells working to fight COVID infections work more efficiently in the presence of oestrogen. This may also be why fewer women than men are likely to die from COVID.

Oestrogen also prevents an enzyme known as ACE (angiotensin-converting enzyme) from causing damage to the heart, lungs, kidneys, nervous system and gut.

What is the evidence showing how oestrogen can help fight COVID-19?

At the time of writing, research into the link between COVID and oestrogen is still emerging because, sadly, women's health is not generally a priority for research. However, an analysis of the electronic health records of nearly 70,000 patients who tested positive for COVID-19, from seventeen countries, showed that women taking replacement oestrogen (HRT) were more than 50 per cent less likely to die from COVID-19 compared to women not taking HRT.[5]

What about 'long COVID'?

Long COVID is defined as when someone has had COVID-19, but is struggling with symptoms for more than four weeks.[6] It has been shown that if a woman is post-menopausal and gets COVID-19, her infection is likely to be more severe.[7]

Women in their early fifties make up the largest group of people who are long-COVID sufferers, and in fact

many symptoms are similar to those of the perimenopause, such as fatigue, joint aches and stiffness, mood
changes, anxiety and brain fog. It is also likely that corona-
virus directly affects the way the ovaries work and produce
hormones.

An online survey of 1,294 women with long COVID
found that three-quarters of respondents reported their
periods had changed since having COVID-19; their
symptoms got worse before or during their periods when
hormone levels were at their lowest.

In the UK, specialist long-COVID clinics have been
established to help people suffering from the long-term
effects of the virus. I believe all women who attend one of
these clinics, or similar clinics worldwide, should be asked
about the possibility of being perimenopausal or menopausal and then offered the appropriate treatment, which
will often include HRT. This is likely to improve many of
their symptoms as well as their future health.

3. Spotlight on Taboo Symptoms

As a healthcare professional with nearly three decades of clinical experience, and as a woman, very little fazes me when it comes to talking about our bodies. Most perimenopausal and menopausal advice focuses on well-known problems such as hot flushes, yet too many symptoms get filed away in the embarrassing or too-difficult-to-discuss box.

I know there are some symptoms – be it vaginal dryness or a low sex drive – that you may feel uncomfortable discussing with your loved ones around the dinner table or with your friends down the pub. You may even feel unable to talk about them with a healthcare professional. I understand that it isn't easy. But in order to tackle these sorts of symptoms with the right treatment you shouldn't be ignoring them, but instead facing them and talking about them.

In this chapter we will lift the lid on these so-called 'embarrassing' symptoms: why they happen, the telltale signs and, crucially, what you can do about them if they happen to you.

Vaginal dryness

Oestrogen is nature's lubricant, which helps keep our vaginas and vulvas healthy. So when oestrogen levels reduce during the perimenopause and menopause, it can thin these tissues, leaving the vagina and the surrounding tissues dry, itchy and inflamed.

Vaginal dryness, 'atrophic vaginitis' or 'vaginal atrophy' are terms often used to describe these symptoms, but the problem actually extends further than that. When most people refer to the vagina, what they often actually mean is the vulva – the term for a woman's external sex organs. The vagina is the short muscular and elastic canal leading from the vulva and the inner and outer lips (known as the labia) to the cervix.

Sex may be painful. However, vaginal dryness is not just a problem for women who are sexually active – it can affect normal everyday activities, such as which clothing or underwear you choose or how long you can sit down for. Riding a bike, or even walking, can be unpleasant and sore.

You might experience intermittent, or even constant, pain at any time of the day, regardless of what you are doing. For other women, discomfort is felt only when the tissues are being stretched, such as during sex or when using tampons. This is because, as well as being drier, the tissue around the vagina has become less flexible and doesn't expand as easily as it did before.

How can it be treated?

Unfortunately these symptoms can persist, or even start, after the end of the menopause, so that's why finding a long-term treatment is so important.

HRT will help to correct the hormone imbalance and will usually ease symptoms (more of this in the next chapter), but a very effective treatment is applying oestrogen directly to the affected area, known as 'local oestrogen'. This is not the same as the oestrogen element of HRT; vaginal oestrogen treatments can be taken safely for a long time and, with no associated risks, can be used alongside HRT.

Local (vaginal) oestrogen is available via a prescription, and there are three main ways to absorb the oestrogen directly from the vagina and surrounding areas:

1. **Pessary**: The most common choice of vaginal oestrogen is to use a pessary (containing an oestrogen called estradiol). This is a small tablet that you insert into the vagina, normally using an applicator. It is administered daily for the first two weeks, and then twice weekly after that. Women usually insert the pessary at night-time so that it can stay in place in the vagina for several hours. If twice weekly doesn't improve the symptoms, it can be used more frequently under advice from your healthcare professional.

   There are also pessaries that contain a more gentle, lower-dose alternative oestrogen called estriol. They look like small waxy bullets. However, they can sometimes result in a discharge when the product dissolves. Women prescribed this are generally advised to use one pessary every night for three weeks, then twice a week thereafter.

Another pessary contains DHEA, a hormone that our body produces naturally. Once positioned in the vagina, the DHEA pessary is converted to both oestrogen and testosterone. It can be used with or without an applicator and the normal dose is one pessary every night.

2. **Cream or gel:** Oestrogen creams are usually inserted inside the vagina every day for two weeks, and then twice weekly after that. An applicator can be used to insert the cream in the vagina, or it can be applied with the fingertips on and around the vulva area as well. There is also a gel, which some women prefer using; this is a lower-dose option and usually comes with an applicator. It is generally used every night for three weeks, then twice a week after that.

3. **Ring:** An oestrogen ring is a soft, flexible silicon ring that you insert inside your vagina. It releases a steady dose of estradiol and is usually replaced every three months. The dose is slightly stronger than the oestrogen pessaries. You can insert the ring yourself or have a healthcare professional do it for you. Women can leave the ring in position to have sex or can remove and reinsert it themselves, if preferred.

4. **Vaginal moisturizers and lubricants:** These products do not contain oestrogen, but help keep the tissues well hydrated and feeling less sore. Moisturizers soothe throughout the day and are

longer-lasting, so you might only need to apply them every two or three days. It is really important that any lubricants or moisturizers you use are balanced to the pH of the vagina and do not cause any irritation or worsening of the symptoms. It is usually worthwhile doing a skin test before use, and you should wash it off immediately if you feel any stinging, burning or itching.

If you know that you have a sensitive vagina or bladder, it is usually best to avoid lubricants containing glycerine or glycols. You should change to another product if you find the lubricant or moisturizer is affecting your vaginal symptoms. Some lubricant and moisturizer companies will send you samples to try, which is a great idea as you may have to try a few brands before you find a product that works for you.

Some lubricants and moisturizers contain perfumes, dyes and flavourings that can be absorbed by the skin, causing allergic reactions and irritation. Certain lubricants contain chemicals to create a tingling/cooling feeling in the genital area and enhance your sexual pleasure. However, these can all make symptoms worse and should usually be avoided.

If you are using condoms for contraception, and you use a lubricant when having sex, make sure it is a water-based lubricant, as this type will not dissolve the latex in the condom.

Urinary, bladder and vaginal problems

It's well known that pregnancy and childbirth, and ageing, can weaken our pelvic floor – the supportive sling of muscles that helps protect our bowel, bladder and uterus and plays a part in sensation during sex. Yet oestrogen plays a part in keeping the pelvic floor healthy, meaning that hormone changes during the perimenopause and menopause can also affect your pelvic floor.

You may find that you experience any of the following symptoms for the first time during your perimenopause or menopause, or that pre-existing issues get worse.

Bladder problems

- **Stress incontinence**: A leakage of urine when coughing or sneezing, lifting or during exercise. Women who experience these problems may be tempted to empty their bladder at more frequent intervals, but this can make the problem worse. In time, your bladder will only hold a small volume of urine and has to be emptied often.
- **Urge incontinence**: When the urge to wee is so strong that leakage happens before you get to the toilet, this is called urge incontinence.
- **Nocturia**: Having to get up at night to go to the toilet.
- **Urinary tract infections (UTIs)**: Some women may also be prone to UTIs, which can result in the need to wee more often, a burning sensation

and abdominal pain. These symptoms can occur without an actual infection and may be a result of low oestrogen levels in the tissues. Some women develop recurrent UTIs, which are UTIs that occurred twice or more in the last six months or more than three times in the last twelve months.

Vaginal problems

- Decreased sensation or pain when having sex
- Prolapse: a feeling of pressure, heaviness or a bulge coming down.

How can these symptoms be treated?

If you are suffering from recurrent UTIs or any of these symptoms it is important to see a healthcare professional for treatment. Incontinence pads and underwear have had a bit of a makeover in recent years, with the more traditional bulky pads being replaced by slimmer, prettier designs. But experiencing leakage, or urinary incontinence, should not be accepted as normal at any point in a woman's life.

The first step is to target your pelvic-floor muscles to regain some strength (see the exercises overleaf). This can be done via pelvic-floor exercises, which, with a little practice, can be performed at home.

If you are concerned about any vaginal or urinary symptoms, please don't suffer in silence. Ask a healthcare professional about a referral to a pelvic-floor physiotherapist, who can assess the extent of your problem and develop an individual plan for you. In addition, replacing the low oestrogen levels in these areas with either vaginal oestrogen or HRT (or often a combination of both) can be really beneficial and can improve these symptoms.

How to carry out pelvic-floor exercises

Nicola Mulkeen is a pelvic-floor physiotherapist who suggests the following exercises.

1. **Sit comfortably with both feet on the floor, and connect with your breathing by taking some deep breaths in and out.**
2. **When you breathe out, squeeze and lift from your bottom to the front where your urethra is, as though you are pulling up a zip. These exercises can take some time to get used to, so try little and often.**
3. **Build up to holding the position for a count of ten seconds, before slowly releasing. Repeat ten times.**
4. **Now try more rapid exercises: quickly lift and squeeze, then release fully. Repeat ten times.**

We do both the slow and fast exercises because the pelvic floor has two types of muscles, called 'slow-twitch muscle fibres' and 'fast-twitch muscle fibres'. With an issue like stress incontinence, we need the muscles to react quickly, so fast exercises can be

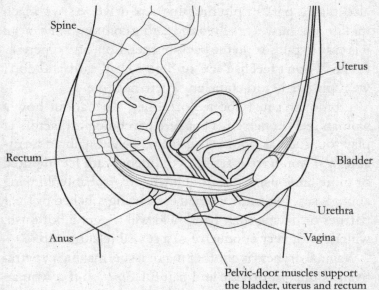

Spine

Uterus

Rectum

Bladder

Urethra

Anus

Vagina

Pelvic-floor muscles support
the bladder, uterus and rectum

The pelvic floor

helpful, while a slower contraction is useful
for endurance and stamina to support us
throughout the day.

Once you have the hang of these exercises,
try to do both versions three to four times a day.

Low sex drive

When oestrogen and testosterone drop, there is a direct
effect on the libido, making arousal difficult. Fatigue can

also play a part in plummeting sex drive. As we reach midlife, our busy work lives and caring commitments mean it is easy to put sex on the back-burner. Lots of women say to me, 'I don't feel like sex' or 'I go to bed early and don't want my partner to come anywhere near me.'

Libido isn't just about hormones – it's about how a woman feels in herself. There are psychological factors at play too, such as poor self-esteem, weight gain and irritability. If you have lost your confidence, are feeling tired or more anxious, the last thing you are probably thinking about is sex. For some women even being touched by their partner or having their hand held will trigger a hot flush, which is not very conducive to a sexual relationship.

Vaginal dryness is another major issue, making penetrative sex uncomfortable and painful. So even if a woman has got a good libido, it might be physically very uncomfortable to have intercourse.

Why sex is still important

In my clinic the majority of women I speak to haven't had intercourse for at least one or two years – not because they don't want to, but because they can't physically. Many women still have a desire to have sex during the menopause. Your midlife is a great time to enjoy sex: children may have moved out, perhaps you have started a new relationship and people generally have a lot more sexual freedom. Plus there are some important health benefits to having regular sex in midlife. People are less likely to develop heart disease, as sex is an aerobic exercise, and it's good for mental health, physical health and your pelvic floor.

How can it be treated?

For the majority of women, having the right dose and type of HRT will help. As vaginal dryness usually lasts beyond the menopause, treatments such as vaginal oestrogen are important for building back up and continuing a healthy sex life. Testosterone in the form of a gel or cream can be used safely alongside HRT or topical oestrogen.

It is also helpful to rethink how we frame sex: it's not just about penetrative sex, but also about having a tactile relationship. Find the right treatment to suit you, and give yourself time: if you haven't had sex for years, it can be daunting to go straight in with intercourse.

> **How to have better sex during your perimenopause and menopause**
> Samantha Evans is a former nurse and co-founder of Jo Divine, an online sex-toy company. She offers the following advice.
>
> The menopause doesn't have to spell the end of your sex life. A 2020 University of Pittsburgh study of 3,200 women aged forty to fifty-five revealed that more than a quarter (27 per cent) rated sexual intimacy as highly important throughout midlife.[1] I am sure the real number

is far higher than this. If your sex life has taken a back seat in recent months and years, try the following to kick-start it.

- Reclaim your intimate health: Sexual health and sexual pleasure go hand-in-hand, so look first to address any physical symptoms you may have. If you are suffering from vaginal dryness, for example, talk to a healthcare professional about treatments such as local oestrogen to ease symptoms.

  A vaginal dilator (once symptoms of vaginal dryness have been adequately treated) can also help to retrain the soft tissues around the vagina and the pelvic-floor muscles. Dilators come in sets, and you start with the smallest first – usually about the size of a tampon – before building up to a large size when it feels comfortable to do so.

  A good-quality lubricant is also a must. Instead of reaching for the first lube you see in the chemist or supermarket aisle, take a close look at the ingredients. Some contain ingredients such as glycerin or sorbitol to make them more slippery, but these can irritate the delicate tissues of the vagina.

  Natural pH-balanced lubricants that are water- or oil-based are a better option, and vaginal moisturizers (available over the

counter) can be used to keep your vagina
moist.

- **Communicate:** It's easy to let our sex lives go,
  so if you have a partner, talk to them. It is so
  important to help them understand why you
  might not want to have sex, or that your menopausal symptoms are making it harder for
  you to become aroused. Give them the opportunity to offer support – you might even find
  that they too have mixed feelings about sex.
- **Go at your own pace:** There is more to
  intimacy than having sex, and holding hands
  and just talking can be a great first step to
  creating that intimacy. A kiss and a cuddle
  don't automatically have to lead to sex,
  unless you want them to.

  Take the focus off penetrative sex and
  incorporate more foreplay, to encourage the
  Batholin's glands near the entrance to the
  vagina to produce the maximum amount of
  natural lubrication. These are a pair of pea-
  sized glands that secrete fluid that acts as a
  lubricant during sex. You could experiment
  with sensual massage; or mutual masturba-
  tion can be a great way to create intimacy.
- **Invest in some goodies** – but make sure you
  do your homework: Regular orgasms will
  help to kick-start your libido. Whether you
  are a seasoned sex-toy user or are trying
  one for the first time, investing in a slim

bullet-style vibrator is a great starting point. You could try it on yourself in the bath or shower, and then with your partner. Think of these products as an investment to reinvigorate and maintain your sex life, rather than as a quick fix. Have some fun!

- **Don't forget to use protection:** You may be entering this phase of your life either newly single or starting a new relationship. If this is the case, you need to think about adequate protection from sexually transmitted infections.

4. HRT and Other Treatment Options to Consider

In the previous chapters we covered the why, the when and the how of all things perimenopause and menopause. We have built up your knowledge base by looking at the causes and symptoms that can affect our well-being. Now it is time to move on to the positive part: the medical treatments that can help to relieve those troublesome symptoms and safeguard your future health.

Finding the right treatment is a huge milestone in your menopause journey, and helping women find a new lease of life after months (or even years) of suffering is what I truly love best about my job as a doctor. In this chapter we will take a closer look at HRT, the most effective treatment to correct your hormone deficiency. We will go into detail about the different types available, the benefits and any risks – and we will bust some myths about HRT along the way.

I have also compiled a list of frequently asked questions about the day-to-day use of HRT by women who come to my clinic, to empower you to get the most out of your treatment. Plus, we will hear about the experiences of women whose quality of life has vastly improved after taking HRT.

We will also cover treatments for women who are unable to take HRT as a first line defence or choose not to take it.

What is HRT?

Hormone replacement therapy does exactly what it says on the tin – it is a treatment to replace the hormones that you are deficient in. As a result, HRT vastly improves your symptoms and helps protect against the long-term health risks of hormone deficiency, including osteoporosis, cardiovascular disease, diabetes and dementia.

What is it made from?

HRT always contains **oestrogen**; it often contains a form of **progesterone**, either known as micronized progesterone or a synthetic progestogen; for some women it also includes **testosterone**. Older forms of HRT contain oestrogens made from a pregnant mare's urine. This is a 'natural' source, and I have known many patients over the years who have taken this type of HRT with no issues at all.

However, menopause medicine has moved on, and the most common type of oestrogen prescribed nowadays is 17 beta-estradiol. This type of oestrogen is available as a patch, gel or spray and is derived from the yam, a root vegetable. It is known as a 'body-identical oestrogen' because, unlike older forms of HRT, it has the same molecular structure as the oestrogen produced by our bodies. I also tend to prescribe a newer type of progesterone called micronized progesterone, which is again derived from yams and is a body-identical hormone.

HRT can be started during the perimenopause and the menopause. The earlier it is taken, the sooner it will work to improve your symptoms and boost your future health.

The different ways you can take HRT

There are dozens of different combinations and dosages of HRT, which may seem daunting at first, but is actually a good thing as it allows flexibility, because each woman's perimenopause and menopause are individual. HRT should always be prescribed by a healthcare professional according to your individual symptoms, age, medical history and personal preferences.

How do I take oestrogen?

Oestrogen is the main component of HRT and can be delivered in various ways, including:

- Skin patch (similar to a small plaster)
- Gel
- Spray
- Oral tablet (although this method is less commonly used these days).

Women who no longer have a uterus (for example, if you have had a hysterectomy) take oestrogen-only HRT and do not usually need to take progesterone. But if you still have a uterus, you need to take a progestogen or progesterone along with the oestrogen, to protect the lining of your uterus. Taking both oestrogen and progesterone (or a progestogen) is known as combined HRT.

What is the difference between oestrogen tablets, patches, gels and sprays?

The patch, gel and spray are known as 'transdermal oestrogen', which gets absorbed directly through your skin into your bloodstream. This means the oestrogen bypasses your liver and causes fewer side-effects; our liver produces clotting factors, which means that if you take a tablet form of oestrogen there is a small increased risk of a blood clot occurring.

Transdermal oestrogen is also suitable if you suffer from migraine, as there is no risk of stroke. The patches result in a more constant amount of oestrogen in your body, so they may be more suitable for women with migraines who are often sensitive to changing oestrogen levels.

How do I take progesterone or progestogen?

The progesterone (or progestogen, a synthetic form of progesterone) component can be delivered as an oral capsule (micronized progesterone) or via the Mirena® coil – a T-shaped device inserted into your uterus that releases a type of progestogen. The coil is also a very effective contraceptive if you need it, and lasts for five years. There are also tablets containing different progestogens.

If you are taking combined HRT, then it is usually preferable to take the oestrogen and progestogen element separately – for example, an oestrogen patch with a micro-nized progesterone capsule.

There are some patches and tablets that contain both oestrogen and a progestogen, but these contain older synthetic forms of progestogen. Synthetic progestogens are more likely to be associated with side-effects such as breast tenderness, bloating and mood swings. Plus using a single combined patch or tablet doesn't allow for flexibility if your dose or method needs to be adjusted.

Why might I need testosterone and how should I take it?

Testosterone can be helpful for some women who are still experiencing symptoms such as fatigue, brain fog or a low sex drive even after taking HRT for a few months.

It is available as a topical cream or gel and while it is currently unlicensed as a treatment for women in the UK, it is widely and safely used by menopause specialists and some GPs. The National Institute for Health and Care Excellence (NICE) has recommended that it is prescribed for menopause-related low sex drive if HRT alone is not effective.[1] Testosterone cream has recently become licensed in Australia, and hopefully it will be licensed in other countries soon.

> ### Four key things to consider when choosing the most appropriate type of HRT
> 1. Your age
> 2. Your medical history

3. **Your symptoms**
4. **Your lifestyle – would a patch suit you better than a daily gel or spray?**

Do I need hormone blood tests to find the right type or dose of HRT?

Not necessarily. A hormone blood test is not usually needed to diagnose the perimenopause and menopause in most women, as this can normally be based on symptoms alone. However, a testosterone blood test is often undertaken before testosterone replacement is started, as it is useful to know what your baseline testosterone level is before beginning treatment. This is not essential, though, because during the perimenopause and menopause testosterone levels will be low.

Another useful blood test is to check the sex-hormone binding globulin (SHBG) level. Using the results of the testosterone and SHBG level tests, a healthcare professional can calculate your 'free androgen index' (FAI). These tests and the FAI should be repeated at regular intervals to ensure that the level remains within the typically female range, so that the unwanted side-effects of testosterone are avoided.

If you are using a transdermal oestrogen patch, gel or spray it can be useful to test your estradiol levels to check that you are absorbing adequate amounts of oestrogen. A low level can indicate that you need a higher dose of oestrogen, or switching the delivery method might be required.

How often do I take HRT?

- If you are using oestrogen-only HRT as a gel or spray, you use it every day. The patches are usually changed twice a week.
- If you are taking combined HRT and your periods have stopped, you use the oestrogen every day and take progesterone every day.
- If you still have periods, even if they are irregular, you use oestrogen every day, and take progesterone alongside it for the last twelve to fourteen days of your menstrual cycle. This will give you a bleed each month and is known as 'monthly cyclical HRT'.
- Another, less commonly recommended type is three-monthly cyclical HRT. You take oestrogen every day and progestogen for two weeks every three months. This will give you a bleed every three months.
- *Note*: Those assigned female at birth who choose to transition with or without testosterone or HRT should speak to a menopause specialist or endocrinologist about what perimenopause and menopause might mean for them.

<u>**Bioidentical HRT: don't believe the hype**</u>
You may have read about 'compounded bioidentical HRT', a treatment offered by some cosmetic and other private clinics and websites.

Not to be confused with 'body-identical HRT', compounded bioidentical HRT is marketed as

a custom-blended product. Some people who prescribe compounded bioidentical HRT claim they are able to determine the precise requirements of each individual woman through a series of complex blood and saliva tests. These test results are used to custom-make tablets, lozenges and creams in doses or preparations that are not routinely available as regulated products.

This is a trend that menopause specialists like me are extremely concerned about. Some of the hormones used in bioidentical products, such as pregnenolone and DHEA, are not approved for women.[2]

In 2019 the British Menopause Society issued a consensus statement that bioidentical products were not regulated, or subject to rigorous safety and efficacy testing, in the same way that conventional HRT is.[3] It also expressed concern that bioidentical products were being prescribed by clinicians who were not experts in the field of the menopause, and that the need for costly tests had never been substantiated through rigorous research and is largely unnecessary.

I know many women who have spent thousands of pounds on these treatments, and some have experienced side-effects such as widespread hair growth on their arms and faces, due to using too high doses of testosterone; and bleeding due to thickening of the lining of the womb because of inadequate progesterone use.

I implore you: please save your money and see your own doctor or a menopause specialist. Approved, registered and regulated body-identical HRT is usually readily available.[4]

You need to be sure that any medication you take – be it for menopause symptoms or otherwise – is safe and appropriate for your individual circumstances.

What are the benefits and the risks of HRT?

I know, from my own personal experience, the transformative effect HRT can have. I am fit and healthy, so I decided to start taking HRT in 2017 to help with my perimeno-pausal symptoms. Within a few months and with some adjustments to the dosage and type, I felt better than I had done in years. The brain fog lifted and my concentration levels and mood improved.

Here are the benefits you can often expect:

- **Relief from your symptoms**: Correcting your hormonal deficiency will greatly ease or stop your symptoms altogether – and for some women this benefit is life-changing. Once you start taking HRT, hot flushes or night sweats should stop within a few weeks, and vaginal and urinary symptoms usually take up to three months (or up to a year in some cases). Your concentration, mood and energy levels should also improve within a few months, as well as your hair and your skin. Put me in a room with ten menopausal women and I could confidently pick out who is taking HRT. I see the effects every day in my clinic: it is visible in a woman's mood, her demeanour, even her skin, and it is so satisfying to witness.

- **Your risk of hormone-related health problems will reduce in the long term:**
  Osteoporosis: Your bones will be protected from weakening due to lack of oestrogen and you will have less risk of fragility fractures when taking HRT.[5]
  Cardiovascular disease: Research has shown that you will be 50 per cent less likely to develop heart problems, stroke or vascular dementia. The benefit is greatest in women who start taking HRT within a decade of their menopause.[6] Interestingly, HRT lowers the risk of cardiovascular disease when started in women aged under sixty more effectively than taking a blood-pressure-lowering medication or a cholesterol-lowering medication.[7]
- **HRT safeguards against other diseases**: Some studies have found that taking HRT can also reduce the risk of developing Alzheimer's disease, osteo-arthritis and depression. Women who take HRT have a lower future risk of Type 2 diabetes and a reduced risk of developing bowel cancer.

What are the risks of taking HRT?

For the majority of women taking HRT, the benefits outweigh any risks. Yet for many years women, healthcare professionals and the media have been given incorrect information about the risks associated with HRT. And too many people focus on the risks rather than the benefits of taking it.

HRT as a treatment has been around for more than fifty years, but in the early 2000s it was the subject of a study that pointed to concerns about an increased risk of breast cancer and cardiovascular disease in women who took combined HRT.[8] However, in this study women used an oral oestrogen and an older type of progestogen. It is also important to look at the profile of the women in this study – they were on average sixty-three years old, and many were overweight or obese or had had heart attacks in the past. Of course it is a perfectly natural reaction to be alarmed when you hear the words 'breast cancer' and 'HRT' mentioned in the same headline. This is the risk factor that women ask me about more than anything else.

More recently, in 2019, research by Oxford University stated that HRT raises the breast cancer risk by one-third.[9] Once again women – understandably – panicked. But as a menopause specialist and a woman who takes HRT, I took a step back and read through the study findings for myself. They arose from an epidemiological study looking at numerous other studies undertaken in the past. It was not a randomized controlled study, which is the gold standard to demonstrate cause and effect. Using observational studies (which have often been undertaken in HRT research) demonstrates an association, but not a cause and effect. It is really important to consider the evidence properly.

My worry is that it is the headlines (and not the drugs themselves) that impact negatively on women's health. Healthcare professionals then won't prescribe HRT to women who stand to benefit, or women decide to come off HRT or not even start it in the first place. This leads to real future health risks.

There are so many different reasons – unrelated to taking HRT – why women develop breast cancer: obesity, not exercising and drinking alcohol are all independent risk factors for developing it. These risk factors are each associated with a higher risk of developing breast cancer than the risk involved in taking any type of HRT.

Numerous perimenopausal and menopausal women I talk to tell me they have put on weight, usually due to a combination of the metabolic changes occurring because of their low oestrogen levels and through comfort-eating. Many women admit they have had to stop exercising as their motivation is low, they are zapped of energy and their joints are stiff and sore. They repeatedly tell me they are drinking more alcohol to 'numb' the symptoms and to try and help them sleep. This means there are millions of women who are increasing their future risk of breast cancer through these lifestyle changes, often without realizing it. Yet they are often too scared to take HRT due to the perceived risks, which are actually lower than the risks created by their lifestyle.

Women who are under fifty-one years and taking any type of HRT do not have an increased risk of developing breast cancer, as they are simply replacing their missing hormones. Women who take oestrogen-only HRT (who have had a hysterectomy in the past) have been shown to have a 25 per cent *lower* future risk of developing breast cancer.[10] Reassuringly, there has never been a study showing that women who take any type of HRT for any length of time have an increased risk of dying from breast cancer.

There is possibly a small increased risk of developing breast cancer for women taking oestrogen with a synthetic progestogen, but this risk is very low – lower than the risk from drinking a moderate amount of alcohol each day. Women who take oestrogen with micronized progesterone have not been shown by any good-quality research to have a higher future risk of developing breast cancer.

Many women who take HRT lose weight, do more exercise and drink less alcohol because they already feel so much better. This means that any potentially increased risk of taking HRT is offset by the improvement in their lifestyle.

HRT and breast cancer: the facts every woman should know

- The baseline risk of breast cancer for women around menopausal age varies from one person to another, according to any underlying risk factors.
- Oestrogen-only HRT is associated with a reduction in a woman's risk of breast cancer.
- Combined HRT containing oestrogen with older types of progestogen has a higher risk compared to taking oestrogen with micronized progesterone.

- The risk of breast cancer with any type of HRT is either not present or is very low.
- There is no increased risk of breast cancer in women under fifty-one years who take any type of HRT.

Clots in the veins (venous thromboembolism)

Taking combined HRT in tablet form carries an increased risk of developing a clot. However, there is no such risk if you use transdermal oestrogen as a patch, cream, gel or spray, as this gets absorbed directly into the bloodstream and bypasses your liver, which produces your clotting factors. Be mindful of other risk factors for clots, including smoking, obesity and a history of clots.

There is a small increased risk of clots for women taking synthetic progestogens as part of their HRT, whereas the micronized progesterone is not associated with an increased risk of clot. Some studies also suggest a small increased risk of stroke from taking oral oestrogen alone, or combined HRT tablets. There is no increased risk of stroke in women using transdermal HRT.

Stephanie, 60

Stephanie, who is now menopausal, started to experience perimenopausal symptoms in her late forties. The perimenopause coincided with a difficult period in her personal life, including the death of a close relative, a marriage break-up and her eighteen-year-old son sustaining life-changing injuries in a car accident.

Stephanie felt anxious, had difficulty concentrating, experienced overwhelming fatigue and irritability, all of which she initially put down to stress. But when she began to have hot flushes, it dawned on her that she might be perimenopausal.

Stephanie told me she decided against 'conventional' HRT after reading articles linking it to blood clots and breast cancer. Instead she bought an unlicensed progesterone cream online, which was marketed as 'bioidentical HRT', believing it was a good 'natural' alternative. She changed her diet, exercised more and was prescribed antidepressants. Her hot flushes reduced, as did her anxiety, but little else.

She still fought fatigue, brain fog and low confidence. Working part-time as a physiotherapist, she found the tiredness and poor concentration were taking their toll. She found herself constantly double-checking her notes and reading articles to ensure she was following best practice, which was tiring in itself. During this time she was also driving her son to numerous medical and legal appointments around the country, and training as an off-road driving instructor (a passion she still enjoyed). Stephanie felt huge anxiety during those appointments and driving assessments.

By 2016 she was considering giving up work, due to

joint pain, fatigue and poor concentration. She decided that HRT (which her mother had taken, while working into her seventies) might be an option.

At her first appointment with me, I talked through Stephanie's health and symptoms and tried to lay her concerns about HRT to rest. I prescribed her body-identical oestrogen in the form of a transdermal gel and micronized progesterone. Within three weeks Stephanie's symptoms had started to ease, and at her follow-up appointment three months later she told me she felt as if she had her old self back.

She does still have some issues sleeping, as well as fatigue and joint pain linked to osteoarthritis, but on the whole she's feeling so much better and more confident.

HRT and the early days: side-effects and getting the right dose for you

We now know what happens to our bodies when our hormone levels are depleted. So reintroducing those hormones your body needs, with HRT, means that you may have some side-effects for a short time while things settle down and until you start feeling your best.

What are the side-effects?

The most common side-effects include some breast discomfort and bleeding. Side-effects are most likely to occur when you first start taking HRT and then usually settle over time. If side-effects have not settled after three to four months, discuss this with your healthcare professional. Your dose or delivery type of HRT might need changing.

What should I do if my symptoms return when I am taking HRT?

Many women need to have some adjustments to their HRT regime, so that both their symptoms and their future health can be optimized. Some women find that simply changing from one type of preparation to another – for example, changing from a tablet to a patch – really improves their symptoms. The 'right' amount of replacement hormones to reduce symptoms as much as possible is not the same from one woman to another. In the same way that people with diabetes need different amounts of insulin, or people with underactive thyroid glands need varying amounts of thyroxine, so oestrogen and testosterone requirements are unique to each woman. Younger women often need higher doses of oestrogen than older women. Different adhesives are used for the patches to stick to the skin; some women find that changing from one type of patch to a different brand improves their absorption of oestrogen through the skin. If a patch is not sticking well or is crinkling, this suggests that you will not absorb the oestrogen properly – you either need to change the patch or change to a different form of oestrogen, such as a gel or spray, instead.

If my symptoms return, does it mean the HRT isn't working?

Many women need their HRT treatment regime altered over time. There may be a noticeable improvement initially, but then not as much as you were hoping for; or there may be a return of some symptoms. You may need a higher dose, or to try a different way of taking the hormone or a different brand. You might benefit from adding in testosterone. Whatever the situation, discuss it with your healthcare professional or see a menopause specialist if you are not satisfied.

Taking HRT: day-to-day practical advice

We help thousands of women every year in my clinic: some are trying HRT for the first time, while others have been taking it for several years. With all the different types and methods available, I want you to feel confident and empowered to take HRT, so here are answers to some of the most common questions that my colleagues and I get asked about using HRT.

Oestrogen gels and sprays

- **Where should I apply the gel?** Licensed directions are to rub the gel into the outside of your upper arm or the inside of your upper thigh. However, some women prefer to rub it in other places, such as all over the thighs, around the shoulder blades or on the lower abdomen. It is fine to do this.

- **Do I have to rub the gel in until it's gone?** It is best to rub it in, rather than leaving it to dry. For most women it is easily absorbed into the skin within a few minutes, so lots of rubbing isn't usually necessary – just the same amount as you would with a moisturizing cream. Once your skin is dry, you can wear clothes and exercise normally. It is generally advisable to wait around thirty minutes before using other creams on the area, such as sunscreen.
- **Where should I use the spray?** Use the spray on the inner part of your forearm. It is advisable to put the oestrogen gel or spray on after having a shower – if this is not possible, try to leave as much time as you can (around an hour is best) between applying the gel or spray and taking a shower, bath or going swimming.
- **Will my partner be affected, if we're intimate?** Wash your hands after applying the gel or spray, and you should leave around an hour before anyone else touches the area where you applied it, to ensure it has been fully absorbed.
- **Can I split the gel or spray dose between morning and night, or does it have to be used all at once?** The most common dose for oestrogen gels or sprays is between two and four pumps a day. Normally, if you need more than this amount, it is preferable to divide the doses between use in

the morning and in the evening. Some women need higher quantities than this, and your doctor will advise you about this if you need more.

Oestrogen patches

- **Where do I apply the patches?** They should be stuck onto the skin below your waist. Most women stick them to the skin on their bottom or upper thigh. If they are not sticking on well, consider changing the brand of patch, as different manufacturers use different adhesives. Some women find wiping their skin with surgical spirit before applying the patches helps them to stick better.
- **Can I shower when wearing patches?** The patches usually stick on well and stay in place in the shower, bath or when exercising.

I take combined HRT: should I take progesterone separately or at the same time as the oestrogen?

The time when you take or use the oestrogen is entirely up to you. However, I usually advise women to take micronized progesterone in the evening, as it has a mild sedative effect and therefore can aid sleep. Also bear in mind that it ideally needs to be taken on an empty stomach (meaning at least an hour after eating).

The key thing to remember is that HRT needs to work around your life. If mornings are hectic and you don't have time to be applying gels or sprays or sticking on patches, do it in the evening. Find a time that works for you. If it becomes part of your daily routine you will be less likely to forget it.

I've been prescribed testosterone cream/gel: how do I apply it?

Rub the testosterone into the lower part of your tummy or on your thigh. You may want to vary the place that you rub the cream or gel every few days to avoid possible growth of a few dark hairs.

Do I need to take a break, if changing from one HRT to another?

There is usually no need to. Do bear in mind that it can take several weeks, or even months, to see an improvement in symptoms or a reduction in side-effects. Some women experience short-term bleeding when increasing the dose of oestrogen.

Can I vary the amount of oestrogen I take throughout the month?

Many women who are perimenopausal notice that their symptoms worsen at certain times of the month. Typically when estradiol levels naturally reduce just before your periods, you can use additional pumps of gel at this time to reduce the exacerbation of symptoms.

What is the maximum amount of HRT I can take?

Women (especially younger women) commonly need to use higher doses of oestrogen than the recommended licensed doses. If a woman is using a higher dose of patch or gel, their estradiol level is usually closely monitored to ensure they are receiving appropriate amounts. It is very safe to use higher doses of oestrogen, and it is important that each woman has adequate oestrogen in her body. If the level is too low, there are future health risks (such as an increased risk of heart disease and osteoporosis) and symptoms are more likely to occur.

Julia, 60

Julia started HRT when she was fifty. After taking it for a decade she made the decision to stop, because she thought that, at sixty, she would be through the effects of the menopause and had been concerned about conflicting reports around the safety of HRT.

The first time she stopped taking it, her symptoms of hot flushes and night sweats came back with a vengeance. She tried to come off HRT twice more, this time reducing the dosage more slowly, but to no avail. Both times her symptoms returned and, at her lowest point, she was experiencing fifteen to twenty hot flushes a day.

Julia turned to herbal medicines, which made no difference. Her family doctor prescribed clonidine, a non-hormone treatment that can be given to treat hot flushes, but this only had a mild effect on her symptoms and led to her feeling very dizzy (a common side-effect). She felt frustrated at the lack of clear advice from her doctor about whether to go back on HRT. All the while she was finding her symptoms debilitating: she wasn't sleeping and felt her sweating was very embarrassing around other people. Julia loved to exercise, but this was off the cards because even walking or using the vacuum cleaner triggered hot flushes.

After a year without HRT, Julia made an appointment to see me. We talked through her medical history, the symptoms that bothered her most, and took a detailed look at the risks and benefits of restarting HRT. It was clear that, for Julia, there were many benefits from taking HRT, including benefits to her future health, and after our appointment she felt more confident and decided to give it another try.

After six weeks she was back on her cross-trainer, her hot flushes reduced to about two per day and her night sweats stopped. Crucially (as I hope you will feel too, after reading the advice in this book), Julia said she felt as if she was back in control of her life.

When do I stop taking HRT?

A lot of women – and healthcare professionals out there – wrongly believe there is a cut-off point for taking HRT. There simply isn't. In fact I've prescribed HRT to a woman in her nineties. It can be continued as long as it is needed, if the benefits outweigh any risks. This usually means for ever, because without HRT our hormone levels are going to be low.

Julia's case underscores how important it is to take an individualized approach to managing menopausal symptoms: your healthcare professional should be looking at your age, your health history, your current symptoms and should take into account your wishes when recommending what treatment to start – or stop.

Other treatments

HRT remains the gold-standard treatment for the perimenopause and menopause. It eases symptoms and helps protect against the long-term health risks of hormone deficiency.

Many women incorrectly think they cannot take HRT. For example, women who have a history of migraines or clots believe they cannot take it, which is incorrect. In addition women with a family history of breast cancer can still usually very safely take HRT.

But what are the options if you are unable, or choose not, to take it?

Antidepressants

Sadly, it is common for women to be inappropriately prescribed antidepressants for menopause-related low mood – despite guidelines from NICE on menopause diagnosis and management clearly stating there is no evidence that antidepressants help with these sorts of mood changes.[11]

However, antidepressants can play a part in managing menopausal symptoms in women who do not take HRT. Antidepressants such as citalopram or venlafaxine, used in low doses, can help to reduce hot flushes and night sweats within a few weeks of starting treatment. They tend to be given to women with a history of hormone-dependent breast cancer, who may not be able to take HRT as a first-line treatment. Side-effects can include a dry mouth and reduced libido.

Clonidine

This is usually a medication for blood pressure but can be given to treat hot flushes. Current guidelines do not recommend that antidepressants or clonidine be given before considering HRT. Clonidine is given in oral-tablet form two or three times a day, and the side-effects can include drowsiness, a dry mouth and depression. In practice, clonidine does not usually help and is not really recommended.

Gabapentin

This is an epilepsy medication used in some countries to treat hot flushes, but it may cause side-effects such as drowsiness and dizziness.

Cognitive behavioural therapy (CBT)

CBT is a talking therapy that has been shown to help with menopausal low mood and anxiety, and even with physical symptoms such as hot flushes and joint pains. It is currently recommended as a treatment for menopause-related low mood and anxiety;[12] see Chapter 6 on menopause and mental health for more details on how it works and how you can access it.

Complementary and alternative medicines

It is very common for women to try herbal medicines or therapies alongside (and sometimes in place of) mainstream medicine to try and alleviate menopause symptoms such as hot flushes and low mood. Below we look at some common medicines and therapies, and at the evidence on their efficacy.

Herbal medicines

There is a very small amount of evidence that taking St John's wort or black cohosh (preparations that are both derived from plants), or isoflavones (derived from soy), can improve hot flushes and night sweats.[13]

To access herbal medicines, you will have to buy preparations in the shops or see a private practitioner. Because there are multiple ways of producing herbal medicines, their quality and potency can vary. If you live in the UK it is worth sticking to products that bear the Traditional Herbal Registration mark (THR). This means that the product conforms to standards around safety and manufacturing.

It is worth remembering that 'natural' does not always mean harmless, and you need to make sure these remedies won't interfere with any other medications you take, or have unwanted side-effects. For example, St John's wort can interfere with breast-cancer drugs such as tamoxifen, and isoflavone supplements are not recommended if you have a history of breast cancer.

Do bear in mind that herbal medicines also won't help protect you against the long-term effects of hormone deficiency, and you should always check with your healthcare professional before using any herbal medicines.

Acupuncture

While there is little scientific evidence about the benefits of acupuncture for menopausal women (in the UK, NICE currently only recommends it as a treatment for migraine and other headaches), many of my patients do find it a beneficial treatment.

Yoga

Yoga is an example of a more holistic treatment. It can be a wonderful way to de-stress and strengthen your bones and muscles through a series of movements (postures).

5. Advice for Women Going through an Early Menopause

The word 'menopause' has become synonymous with midlife. However, menopause in younger women is far more common than most people realize. My youngest patient is only nineteen years old. Around one in every 100 UK women will go through their menopause before their fortieth birthday.[1]

When I was at medical school we were taught that when periods stopped in younger women it was probably down to one of two reasons: mostly likely she was pregnant, or it could be related to an eating disorder. The word 'menopause' was never mentioned as a possible cause. Thankfully, things are changing around menopause awareness, but there is still much more that can be done for women whose menopause starts at a younger age.

The menopause is tough to deal with at the best of times, but in younger women it can be an unexpected and difficult diagnosis to come to terms with. Some women may be planning to have a family in the near future or have started trying already. Discovering that their body is already preparing for menopause can come as a huge blow, and not only are they dealing with troublesome symptoms at a younger age, but also with long-term health risks, because their hormone levels are lower for longer. That is why a prompt diagnosis and treatment are so important.

If you are a woman who thinks you may be going through an early menopause, then this chapter is written especially for you. It includes an overview of potential causes, symptoms and long-term health implications of the menopause at a younger age.

We will also run through the treatment options to maintain your current and future health and to help you stay happy, healthy and live your life the way you want to.

What is an early menopause?

As we now know, the average age of the menopause in the UK is fifty-one, with perimenopausal symptoms often starting at around forty-five years of age. When we talk about menopause in younger women, two key definitions come into play:

1. **Early menopause**, which applies to women who are aged forty to forty-five and who have not had a period for twelve consecutive months.
2. **Premature ovarian insufficiency (POI)**, which refers to women who go through the menopause before the age of forty.

Why do some women go through the menopause earlier than others?

For the vast majority of women the underlying cause is not known. However, it can be due to one of the following:

- **Cancer treatments**: Radiotherapy, particularly to your pelvic area, and chemotherapy can cause an early menopause. This is covered in more detail in Chapter 10 on menopause and cancer.
- **Surgery**: An operation to remove your ovaries, known as an oophorectomy, leads to POI. And so too can a hysterectomy (where your uterus is removed), even if your ovaries are not removed. This is because it is common for oestrogen levels to fall at an earlier age after a hysterectomy.
- **Autoimmune disease, such as thyroid or adrenal problems**: This is where your immune system (which normally protects your body from infection) mistakenly attacks body tissues. Autoimmune disease is responsible for about one in twenty cases of POI.
- **Genetic conditions**: The most common of these is Turner syndrome, where one of the female chromosomes is missing. POI due to a genetic condition is usually more common if you have family members with POI, or if POI starts at a very early age.

Symptoms of early menopause and POI

The symptoms of early menopause or POI can be similar to those of women who go through their menopause in later life, including low mood, brain fog, fatigue and hair and skin changes. Yet many younger women may be in early menopause without realizing it. Symptoms can come and go as hormone levels fluctuate, and a significant

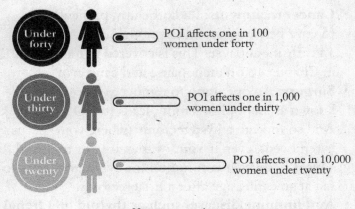

POI affects one in 100 women under forty

POI affects one in 1,000 women under thirty

POI affects one in 10,000 women under twenty

How common is premature ovarian insufficiency?

proportion of women (about 10–15 per cent) won't have any symptoms at all.

That is why tracking any period changes can be very useful, as this can often be the first sign. You might experience a change in flow, and your periods will become less frequent, before stopping completely. However, for about one in ten young women with POI, their periods never start in the first place.

It is so important that if you have irregular periods, or your periods have stopped, you talk to a healthcare professional, regardless of your age.

How is POI or early menopause diagnosed?

The process of diagnosis tends to be more detailed for younger women than for those who go through the menopause at the usual, later age. This is because the health implications of an early menopause are so much greater.

If you have had both your ovaries removed, then you won't need any tests to confirm your diagnosis. Otherwise, a healthcare professional should be talking to you about any symptoms and about your own and your family's medical history. It is likely that you will need to have a blood test to measure your FSH levels. If these are raised, then it is very probable that you are menopausal. This test should be repeated four to six weeks later to confirm the diagnosis, because your FSH levels change at different times during your menstrual cycle. However, as FSH levels can fluctuate so much, a normal FSH level does not exclude POI as a diagnosis.

You should also have a bone-density (DEXA) scan to check the density of your bones, as low levels of oestrogen increase the risk of developing osteoporosis. You may be offered other blood tests to check your glucose level, thyroid and to test for coeliac disease too, as these can be associated with POI in some women. If you are under thirty-five, you may be offered a blood test to check your chromosomes, to determine whether a chromosomal problem is causing POI.

If it is unclear whether you are in an early menopause, you should be referred to a healthcare professional who specializes in menopause or reproductive medicine to confirm your diagnosis. Please keep going until you have a firm answer, because starting the right treatment promptly is so important to your current and future health.

Three key questions to ask your doctor

- Can you explain what has caused my early menopause/POI and why it has happened to me?
- Are there any health risks associated with untreated early menopause or POI?
- What is the impact on my fertility?

Hayley, 39

Hayley started her periods when she was twelve years old, but within a year they had stopped. She was struggling to concentrate in lessons at school during the day, and at night she was waking up dripping with sweat.

Hayley confided in her mother about how she was feeling, and they made an appointment with her GP. Hayley was referred to a consultant gynaecologist for blood tests and an ultrasound. It emerged that her uterus was smaller than average and she only had one ovary; two weeks later she was given the news that she had gone through the menopause.

Looking back, Hayley says she didn't really understand the significance of the news and couldn't appreciate why her mother was so upset. Hayley was just fourteen years old when she found out that she had been through the menopause. She was prescribed HRT, but this was the first and last time she saw her consultant. No guidance or follow-up appointments were offered, and she was left to 'get on with it'.

When the type of HRT she took was discontinued a few years later, Hayley only found out when she went to the pharmacist to pick up her usual prescription. She managed to make an appointment with her GP the next day and was prescribed a different brand, but this didn't suit her and her symptoms returned. Her doctor then prescribed an alternative, and although this time it suited her more, Hayley still did not feel completely better.

She grew up disliking her appearance and felt insecure. She struggled with relationships, as she knew that one day she would have to tell partners about her menopause. A lack of awareness about POI meant that to this day even friends do not understand. In the absence of much-needed support from healthcare professionals, Hayley had to learn how to cope alone.

She has decided to speak out about her experiences to try and raise awareness of POI. Quite rightly she says she should have been given more advice on what was happening to her body, and more input in her treatment.

Hayley's story saddens me so much because she has had to struggle on for so long without adequate help, advice or treatment. She feels that even now – more than two decades on from her diagnosis – there needs to be more tailored information for young women going through the same thing. Her story will resonate with so many women who are neglected during their perimenopause and menopause. With increasing awareness of the symptoms that can occur during the menopause and of the health risks of the menopause, women deserve better treatment. It is essential that all women can access evidence-based health and treatment for their menopause.

How an early menopause impacts on your future health

Oestrogen is hugely important to so many functions in our body, but four key areas that are impacted the most when our oestrogen levels fall at a younger age are: our bone health, our brain health, our cardiovascular health and our sexual health. Many women with POI usually benefit from testosterone too.

1. **Bone health:** Oestrogen helps to protect our bones and maintain bone density, so falling oestrogen levels earlier than the average age of the menopause means that younger women are at increased risk of developing osteoporosis.[2]
2. **Brain health:** Our brains need oestrogen on board to help with memory, mood and concentration. Research has shown that women who go through the menopause at an earlier age are at increased risk of dementia in later life. Oestrogen and testosterone are also important for our mood. It can be socially isolating to go through the menopause at

a younger age, and I certainly see people in my clinic who have felt unable to talk to their friends or peers about what they are going through.

3. **Cardiovascular health**: Oestrogen helps protect our arteries and lower cholesterol, and an early menopause puts women at increased risk of cardiovascular disease. A 2019 study found that women under forty who experienced premature menopause were nearly twice as likely to have a non-fatal cardiovascular event, such as a heart attack, angina or stroke, before the age of sixty.[3]

4. **Sexual health**: Testosterone production decreases by more than 50 per cent in women with POI, which can affect libido and mood as well as memory and concentration.

What about my fertility?

It is important to realize that for a lot of women with early menopause or POI, it doesn't necessarily mean they are infertile. Unlike menopause in older women, the ovaries often don't completely stop working in women with POI.

Ovarian function can fluctuate over time, occasionally resulting in a period, ovulation or even pregnancy. This intermittent return of ovarian function can result in about 5–10 per cent of women being able to conceive. Taking HRT can actually improve fertility in some women and is usually safe to continue if you become pregnant while taking it. If having children is something you were considering now or in the future, ask about a referral to a fertility specialist to discuss your options.

And if you are prescribed HRT, bear in mind that we have had a few cases at the clinic where women with POI have been delighted to fall pregnant while taking it. But if getting pregnant is not part of your plan, then make sure you are using adequate contraception.

Treatment options: HRT and the combined oral contraceptive pill

Speak to a healthcare professional about deciding on the right treatment for you, taking into account your symptoms, your medical history and your existing conditions.

Unless there is a medical reason why you can't take hormones, or you don't want to, this is by far the most appropriate treatment. When treating women going through an early menopause we want to do two things: try to ease their current symptoms and, crucially, prevent future damage from not having enough hormones.

Treatment for POI or early menopause usually involves taking combined HRT or the combined oral contraceptive pill. Both treatments contain oestrogen and a progestogen (or progesterone) and replace the hormones that you are deficient in. HRT is safer and has more evidence to support improving your future health, such as lowering your future risk of heart disease and osteoporosis. Generally speaking, the younger you are, the higher dose of hormones you need to correct the deficiency.

If you are diagnosed with early menopause or POI it is important that you take hormones until at least the age of fifty-one, the natural age of menopause. This will replace hormones that your body would otherwise be making up to the age of your natural menopause, and offer protection from osteoporosis and other conditions that can develop after menopause. Usually women continue to take HRT after this age, and the majority of women continue taking HRT for ever.

HRT or the combined oral contraceptive pill?

The hormones delivered via HRT using body-identical oestrogen, progesterone and testosterone provide hormones that are the same molecular structure as the hormones we are replacing in our bodies. The method and dosage can also be changed very easily.

Often younger women may be more comfortable with the combined oral contraceptive pill because it is familiar, and offers contraceptive benefits if there is a possibility that you could become pregnant naturally and you do not wish that to happen. However, using oestrogen and testosterone with the Mirena® coil is usually the preferable way of taking HRT if you need contraception. But the contraceptive pill is not suitable if you are aged over thirty-five years and a smoker, or if you have cardiovascular disease or a history of blood clots, stroke or migraines.

Key points about these treatments:

- Both treatments should improve your symptoms.
- For the majority of women who start taking HRT for POI, the benefits of HRT far outweigh any risks.
- There is more evidence to support taking HRT to improve your future health than taking the contraceptive pill.
- Many women with POI benefit from taking testosterone too.
- HRT is better for your blood pressure than the combined oral contraceptive pill.
- HRT is not a contraceptive – unless you are using the Mirena® coil.[4]

Other treatments

Testosterone

Not all women will need testosterone, but talk to your healthcare professional if you find that HRT or the combined contraceptive pill alone is not helping with symptoms such as low libido, low mood, lack of energy or concentration.

Treatments for vaginal dryness and urinary symptoms

Local oestrogen in the form of a cream, gel, vaginal tablet or ring inserted into the vagina can help ease symptoms.

This can be safely given with HRT. Another option for dryness is vaginal moisturizers and lubricants during sex, which can be used with local oestrogen treatments.

Cognitive behavioural therapy (CBT)

It is quite common to have feelings of low mood or anxiety following a diagnosis of early menopause or POI. It is a huge life change and may be happening many years before you expected it. CBT may be beneficial and is recommended as a possible treatment.

Lifestyle changes

Maintaining a good diet and a healthy lifestyle, in conjunction with the right treatment, is so important, regardless of the age at which you go through the menopause.

6. Menopause and Mental Health

If I stood outside my clinic today and surveyed passing members of the public about telltale signs of the menopause, I would expect the majority would know about hot flushes. Yet I would wager that very few would be aware of the enormous impact our perimenopause and menopause can have on our mental health and well-being. The widespread lack of understanding around the effect of hormones on our mood means that menopause-related psychological symptoms can be misdiagnosed – or often missed completely.

For most women the menopause coincides with one of the most hectic periods of our lives: we are probably established in our career and are juggling work with family, and may be supporting teenagers or have other caring responsibilities. It is easy to put symptoms like irritability and sudden outbursts down to tiredness, or to blame rising anxiety on worrying about work, ageing parents or teenage children. And for those women who do seek help from their doctor, many will be offered antidepressants, despite the fact that these simply don't work for menopause-related low mood.

We urgently need to educate ourselves about why the perimenopause and menopause can have such a huge impact on our mental health. The highest rate for suicide among females is in the fifty to fifty-four age group,[1] precisely the average age of menopause. Sadly, I believe this is no coincidence.

Looking after our mental health is not an optional extra. In this chapter we will look at how fluctuating hormones affect our mood, the treatments that can help – and the ones that won't – and some simple strategies to safeguard your mental health and well-being.

The link between the perimenopause and menopause and our mood

Falling oestrogen, progesterone and testosterone can impact on our brains and, as a result, on our mood.

Oestrogen stimulates serotonin, a mood-boosting chemical that regulates our state of mind and anxiety. Oestrogen also plays a role in the production of endorphins, the brain's 'feel-good' chemicals.

Progesterone is a natural sedative that relaxes our brains and bodies. During the perimenopause and menopause our bodies will try to compensate for declining progesterone levels by releasing the stress hormones cortisol and adrenaline, which can make us feel anxious and irritable. This can happen very quickly, and can therefore trigger extreme emotions or outbursts.

Testosterone also often works in our brains to improve mood, energy and motivation.

Then, of course, there is the knock-on effect of physical perimenopausal and menopausal symptoms. If you are worn out by frequent hot flushes or aches and pains, feel frustrated by your itchy skin or can't concentrate during an important meeting, you are bound to feel low.

The crucial difference between clinical depression and menopause-related mood changes

Typically clinical depression is a continuous feeling of sadness, with symptoms such as feeling hopeless, tearful, anxious or irritable. It can affect sleep, appetite and sex drive. In severe cases, people with clinical depression have suicidal thoughts or ideas about harming themselves.

Perimenopause- and menopause-related mental-health symptoms can include:

- Mood swings and low mood
- Low energy and fatigue
- Feelings of guilt
- Irritability, anger, rage
- Low self-esteem and feelings of worthlessness
- Reduced interest in socializing, feeling isolated
- Increased anxiety and panic attacks
- Disrupted sleep and insomnia
- Lack of libido and reduced sexual enjoyment
- Problems with memory and concentration
- Agitation.[2]

While symptoms of clinical depression and menopause-related mood changes can overlap (for example, anxiety and feeling irritable), one crucial difference is that where clinical depression is a continuous feeling of low mood lasting weeks or months, mood changes due to the perimenopause or menopause tend to fluctuate. Often women know that their symptoms are different from symptoms of clinical depression. It can be common for feelings of sadness, anxiety or even flashes of rage to come and go.

Perimenopausal women will often describe how they feel absolutely fine one week, only to be floored by anxiety the next. This is because these mood changes may be most severe when our oestrogen levels are at their lowest. Oestrogen levels rise during the first half of the menstrual cycle and fall during the second half, meaning that women who experience pre-menstrual syndrome (PMS) usually have mood swings or feel teary in the days before their period. So when oestrogen levels fluctuate, particularly during the perimenopause, it is understandable that you will find your mood is negatively affected.

Keep a mood diary

If you are unsure of the root cause of your mood changes, try keeping a brief mood diary or record how you feel on my free menopause Balance app.

Jot down or record how you feel each day (happy, sad, anxious, angry, irritated) and when you have your periods. This will help you and your healthcare professional to determine whether your hormones are affecting your mood. If you have had PMS or post-natal depression in the past, you may find you are more likely to experience mood changes during your perimenopause and menopause, as you are more sensitive to hormone changes.

How to tackle mood changes

Talk through your full range of symptoms with your healthcare professional to find the right treatment to tackle your mood changes.

Explore HRT treatment options

Ideally you should look to replace oestrogen (and possibly also testosterone) and balance your hormones with HRT. If you take HRT, you should see your mood improve within a few months. If you find it is not working, talk to your healthcare professional about altering the dosage or method of HRT. If it still doesn't improve, you could discuss the option of a testosterone cream or gel. Not everyone will need or benefit from this, but many of my patients find it beneficial for their mood.

Note: Your mental health is extremely important. If you don't feel you are getting the help you need, please persevere. Ask for a second opinion or request to see someone else.

Why antidepressants are not always the answer
Let me be clear: antidepressants work well as a treatment for people with clinical depression. In my many years as a GP, I have seen thousands of women and men with clinical depression who have benefited from antidepressants. Likewise, I have treated thousands of menopausal women with low moods who are

not clinically depressed. Menopause guidelines are very clear: antidepressants should not be given as first-line treatment for low mood associated with the menopause,[3] because there is no evidence that they will help.

Yet too many menopausal women are still being incorrectly offered antidepressants by their doctor. A 2019 study of nearly 3,000 women in the UK by my non-profit organization Newson Health Research and Education showed that 66 per cent of women said they had been offered or given antidepressants for low mood associated with their menopause. This usually happens when mental-health symptoms are being looked at in isolation, and not in conjunction with other symptoms, such as joint pains, vaginal dryness or fatigue.

Antidepressants work by increasing levels of the chemicals serotonin and noradrenaline in our brain, which are linked to mood and emotions. But what antidepressants won't do is address your menopause-related hormone deficiency in the way that HRT does. Antidepressants, when prescribed inappropriately, could cause side-effects such as blunted mood and reduced sex drive. They will not reduce the future risk of diseases such as heart disease and osteoporosis in the same way that taking HRT does.

Research has also shown that if women are given HRT when they are perimenopausal, this can reduce the incidence of clinical depression developing in the first place. In my experience, many of the women who take HRT and have been incorrectly given antidepressants in the past find their depressive symptoms improve, to the extent that they can reduce and often stop taking their antidepressants.

Cognitive behavioural therapy (CBT)

CBT is a talking therapy that can help you manage your problems by changing the way you think and behave. It is widely used for a range of physical and mental-health issues, including anxiety and depression, insomnia and chronic fatigue syndrome.

- **How can it help me?** CBT is recommended in menopause guidelines as a treatment to alleviate menopause-related low mood or anxiety.[4] The core model of CBT focuses on the here and now, examining an event or difficult situation and looking at how you respond to it. CBT teaches you how to recognize unhelpful behaviours (such as negative thoughts and emotions) and shows how you can react to challenges in a more positive way.
- **How do I access CBT?** CBT is a well-established treatment that is used worldwide, so speak to your medical team about how you can access it. If you

Situation: → **Thought:** → **Emotion:** → **Behaviour:**
something happens | the situation is interpreted | a feeling occurs as a result of the thought | an action in response to the emotion

The theory behind cognitive behavioural therapy

live in the UK you can ask your GP to refer you to an NHS psychological-therapies service or you can refer yourself directly. There can be a wait for a place on a course to become available, so going private can be quicker. The British Association for Behavioural and Cognitive Psychotherapies has a list of accredited CBT therapists (www.cbt-registeruk.com). It is also worth checking with your workplace human-resources department, as companies can sometimes offer access to CBT as part of their employee assistance programmes.

Mindfulness

This is the practice of being in the moment and paying attention to your thoughts, your surroundings and the sensations of your breathing and your body. With mindfulness, the aim is not to empty your mind of worries, but to notice them, acknowledge them and visualize worries as passing through.

- **How can it help me?** There is growing evidence
  that mindfulness can help us all deal with issues such
  as stress, anxiety, depression and insomnia. Specific
  research has also been carried out looking into
  the effects of mindfulness on menopause-related
  symptoms. A 2019 review found that psychological interventions like mindfulness and CBT can
  help with symptoms such as hot flushes, irritability,
  forgetfulness and joint pain.[5] And a study involving 1,750 women aged forty to sixty-five found that
  those who practised mindfulness regularly had lower
  levels of irritability, depression and anxiety.[6]
- **How can I access mindfulness sessions?** Mindfulness can be done alone at home, but there are
  some structured courses available on the NHS if
  you live in the UK, so speak to your GP about
  these. As with CBT, waiting lists can be long and
  availability varies. And wherever you live, you could
  opt for paid, private sessions. Check out the British
  Association for Mindfulness-Based Approaches
  (www.bamba.org.uk) for a list of qualified mindfulness teachers. There are also some easy-to-use apps
  like Headspace (www.headspace.com) and Calm
  (www.calm.com) which offer guided meditation and
  relaxation exercises.

Mindfulness exercise: body scan

This is a mindfulness exercise that is suitable for beginners.
Try and set aside about fifteen minutes for this exercise,

picking a time of day when you know you won't be disturbed – and remember to set your phone to silent.

1. Lie on your back on the floor or on your bed, making sure you feel warm and comfortable.
2. Extend your legs and rest your arms beside your sides, with the palms of your hands facing up.
3. Start by concentrating on your breathing – breathing deeply in through the nose and out through the mouth. Do this for two minutes.
4. Then, slowly and deliberately, focus your attention on each part of your body, starting at your toes and slowly moving up to your head.
5. Pay attention to the sensations or emotions you feel in each part of your body.
6. If your thoughts drift away, notice them and gently guide them back to your body. You should feel calmer after this exercise, but if you find your mind drifting, keep at it – it will get easier with practice.

Kate, 55

A few years ago, when she was in her late forties, Kate began to experience perimenopausal symptoms. She would occasionally worry about things, but was able to cope when challenges arose.

This changed when her perimenopause began. Around the time her period was due each month, she began to feel consumed by feelings of anxiety, exhaustion and worsening PMS. Bouts of inexplicable anxiety and panic attacks made her feel low and affected her self-esteem. There was no telling when the anxiety would strike: once she was at a supermarket checkout and just wanted to run out. She also started having night sweats, which made it hard to sleep, and had a series of urinary tract infections (UTIs), which she had never had before.

Seeking help for her anxiety and other symptoms, Kate went to see her doctor. HRT was discussed, but only as an option for further down the line. Instead Kate focused on diet and lifestyle changes. She ate more healthily, took supplements, cut down on her alcohol intake and upped her levels of exercise. Things did improve a little, but over time her periods became more erratic and Kate started to experience fatigue and brain fog, which made it hard to concentrate. She found herself snapping at her two children for no reason, experienced bouts of intense rage aimed at no one in particular, and her libido started to suffer. Kate says the final straw was when she began to suffer joint pains, particularly in her feet, which made it difficult for her to exercise.

When Kate came to see me, we went through her long list of symptoms and talked through her individual risks and the benefits of HRT. I prescribed a combined HRT, in the form of oestrogen gel and micronized progesterone, coupled with a small amount of testosterone cream. The testosterone has helped with her sense of well-being, her physical strength and her libido. In combination with the oestrogen gel, it has got rid of the 'brain fog'.

In the eighteen months since she started HRT, Kate has no longer had panic attacks, she has more energy and her self-esteem has been restored. Most of the physical aches and pains have gone, and her brain fog has lifted. She says she now has a renewed sense of purpose, and her only wish is that she had started taking HRT earlier.

Further strategies to boost your mental health

Women often tell me how their low moods make them shut the door on everyone and everything, including those closest to them. Others feel a tremendous amount of guilt about how their moods or outbursts have affected those around them.

Communicate

You do not have to carry this burden alone. Talking to a healthcare professional and getting the right treatment is an incredibly important step, but you also need to let your friends, family and trusted work colleagues in. It is difficult for loved ones to see you going through these physical and emotional challenges. I have seen partners who have accompanied women to my clinic in tears because they don't know how to help.

Tell them how you are feeling; educate them about how your hormones are affecting you. Is there something they can do to help? Do certain tasks or situations make your anxiety worse, and could they be offloaded onto someone else?

Get moving

With the right treatment you should see your energy levels improve and your physical symptoms subside. If you don't exercise regularly, now would be a great time to build some exercise into your routine. Exercise releases feel-good endorphins and has a multitude of health benefits, from promoting better sleep to protecting your heart and bones.

See Chapter 8 on exercise for some inspiration. But if you haven't exercised in a while, don't get too hung up about how much exercise you do and how often; start with something gentle, like walking, and take it from there.

Set aside time for self-care

When you are coping with low mood and anxiety there can be an all-pervading sense of negativity, from thoughts of 'I can't cope' to catastrophizing about the worst thing that might happen. So give yourself a break – literally. Many of us find it hard to relax when our lives are so hectic, but it is incredibly important. Many of my patients find that aromatherapy can lift their mood and aid relaxation. You can use a few drops of essential oil diluted with a carrier oil during massage or add a little to a bath. Book in time in advance to do something you enjoy – be it spending time alone catching up with a box set, exercising or calling a friend.

7. Menopause and Sleep

Having trouble sleeping? Then you are in good company. Almost every single woman who comes through the door of my clinic complains of being tired due to poor sleep.

Exhausted-looking patients tell me of waking several times due to night sweats, often even waking before the actual sweating occurs. Others are woken by nocturia (the night-time urge to wee). Many women wake several times, especially in the early hours, even if they don't have night sweats. And then there are women who go to bed nice and early, only to find it impossible to switch off, sitting bolt upright for hours as their partner snores happily next to them.

The power of hormones on sleep should not be underestimated, and during our perimenopause and menopause good-quality sleep is more important than ever. Research shows that sleep problems are more common as women enter the perimenopause and menopause.[1] So in this chapter we will look at the reasons why so many of us are plagued by poor sleep. We will also look at the treatments to help correct hormonal issues, and at some strategies to help send you off to the Land of Nod.

The science behind sleep

Sleep is central to our general health and well-being. It reduces inflammation, helps to promote wound-healing and repair in our bodies and supports our immune system. Sleep is also crucial for brain health – a disturbed night's sleep affects our short-term memory and reaction time. In terms of mental health, it helps safeguard against stress and depression.

Sleep also helps us control our blood-sugar levels and maintain a healthy weight. Studies have shown that sleep-deprived people have lower levels of leptin, a hormone that makes you feel full, and higher levels of ghrelin, a hormone that stimulates hunger.

When it comes to defining a good night's sleep, people become fixated on how many hours of sleep they get a night. However, there is no standard definition of what constitutes 'normal' sleep. The amount of sleep needed to ensure good health varies from person to person[2] and depends on factors such as our age.

What is important is sleep quality. When we sleep, we go through several rounds of a sleep cycle, with each cycle split into a number of stages. These stages are important in helping our brain and body recover and develop, and so interrupted sleep – or failing to fall asleep in the first place – can impact on our physical and mental health.

<u>What is the secret to good-quality sleep?</u>
America's National Sleep Foundation has identified the four key determinants of quality sleep:

1. **The vast majority of time in bed should be spent sleeping (at least 85 per cent of the total time)**
2. **Falling asleep in thirty minutes or less**
3. **Waking up no more than once per night**
4. **Being awake for twenty minutes or less, after initially falling asleep.**[3]

How do the perimenopause and menopause affect sleep?

For the majority of my patients it is dealing with the impact of menopausal symptoms that causes sleep problems. And it should come as no surprise that night sweats and hot flushes come top of the list – and I know, from personal experience, just how disruptive they can be. Before the penny dropped that I was perimenopausal and I began taking HRT, I experienced horrendous night sweats nearly every night for months. I would wake up in the middle of the night drenched in sweat and would often have to change my sheets and pyjamas. I was also waking up at other times when I wasn't having night sweats; just lying in bed, knowing I would be tired the following day but finding it impossible to get back to sleep.

Other symptoms that interfere with sleep include joint aches and pains, and urinary problems such as recurrent UTIs and nocturia. Women who suffer from these symptoms say they cause them to wake during the night or make it hard to fall asleep in the first place.

Psychological symptoms linked to the menopause can also play havoc with our sleep. Many women with low mood or anxiety tell me that their mind races as soon as their head hits the pillow, or that they wake early, worrying about work or home life.

In addition, our hormones play an important role in supporting our brain to ensure sleep quality and duration. Oestrogen can help our brains process serotonin – a chemical building block for melatonin, a hormone that helps to regulate our sleep/wake cycle. Progesterone can also be beneficial for sleep. It increases production of a chemical in our brains called GABA (gamma-aminobutyric acid), which calms our brain and relaxes our body ready for sleep. Low GABA activity can be linked to insomnia and poor sleep, stress and poor concentration, while low testosterone levels have also been linked to sleep problems.

Correcting the hormone deficiency should also improve aches and pains and should see urinary problems settle down. Again, if you are suffering from recurrent UTIs you should always consult a healthcare professional in case it is not linked to the menopause.

What you can do about it

The first step you can take is to talk to a healthcare professional about treatment for your symptoms.

Correct your hormone deficiency

Studies have shown that HRT improves sleep quality, enables falling asleep, decreases night-time wakefulness and reduces symptoms.[4] Adequate levels of oestrogen can often make a dramatic improvement to sleep. Women often notice that they can fall asleep quicker and wake fewer times in the night.

Many women take micronized progesterone as the progesterone part of their HRT. As mentioned in Chapter 4 on HRT, micronized progesterone is a natural sedative so it can cause drowsiness, which is a beneficial side-effect for many women who are having trouble sleeping.

Skip 'catch-up' sleep in favour of a consistent bedtime

There is nothing worse than spending the night tossing and turning and then having to get up and face the day. And while our bodies can cope with an occasional night of disrupted sleep, if you find yourself in a cycle of poor sleep, then it needs to be addressed.

So many of us try to repair a bad night by having an early night the following evening to catch up on lost sleep. We also often try and offset poor sleep during the working week by sleeping in later at the weekend. But trying to catch up in these ways can be counterproductive.

Head off to bed too early and you will probably lie there feeling frustrated, and it will lead to you seeing your bed as a place where you feel restless, not rested. And while of course it is a lovely treat, I'm afraid that weekend lie-ins won't magically make up for night after night of poor sleep.

One 2019 sleep study looked at the sleep of healthy adults, dividing them into three groups. One group was allowed plenty of time to sleep – nine hours each night for nine nights. The second was allowed five hours per night over that same period. The third slept no more than five hours nightly for five days, followed by a weekend when they could sleep as much as they liked, before returning to two days of restricted sleep. People in the weekend catch-up group gained weight and had a lower insulin sensitivity, a risk factor for Type 2 diabetes.[5]

Consistency, not catching up, is key. That means going to bed and getting up at the same time, even at weekends (sorry!). Doing this will set your body's internal clock, known as the circadian rhythm. Our circadian rhythms are individual, so it is important to work out the optimal time for you. If you naturally wake up early, then go to bed early, and vice versa. Make sure you set an alarm to help establish the routine.

Write your worries away

Even if you don't suffer from physical symptoms such as night sweats or urinary issues, psychological menopause symptoms can be incredibly disruptive to sleep. Patients tell me they will wake in the middle of the night with their minds racing about home, work or situations beyond their control. This can leave them feeling overwhelmed, anxious and unable to get back to sleep.

Kathryn Pinkham is an NHS insomnia specialist and founder of the Insomnia Clinic. She suggests setting aside twenty minutes each day to write down anything that is playing on your mind – be that a to-do list, random thoughts or 'what if'-type worries. Writing them down acknowledges them and, if done regularly, they are less likely to pop into your head just before falling asleep or in the middle of the night.

I have learned over the years, from talking to my patients, that there will be certain situations or environments that we cannot change. However, what we can change is the way we deal with them, even if it is just by acknowledging that they exist.

Wendy, 48

Wendy had menopausal symptoms for two years before coming to my clinic. She explained that she was fatigued, found it difficult to concentrate and felt as if she was permanently on the verge of coming down with a cold.

Sleep was a key issue. Despite going to bed at the same early hour as her eight-year-old son, when she woke up every morning Wendy wasn't refreshed – she felt shattered. She explained that she occasionally had night sweats that woke her up. She usually went to sleep very quickly, but then woke up at various times of the night (and early in the morning) and really struggled to get back to sleep. She never woke up feeling refreshed.

The crushing tiredness and lack of energy were impacting on her career. She described how writing an important business plan at work 'nearly broke' her because she just couldn't concentrate. She was having frequent days off work, making the excuse that she had migraines, as she could not explain to her boss that she was simply tired.

It was clear, taking into account Wendy's symptoms and health history, that she would benefit from taking HRT. After I worked out the right dosage and type of HRT for her, Wendy's symptoms soon improved. She found that, within a few days of taking HRT, her sleep really improved and she rarely woke up during the night. This meant that her tiredness subsided and she could concentrate at work.

Wendy's admission about going to bed early to 'catch up' with sleep goes to show that an early night, or sleeping in later, is no guarantee of a good night's sleep. Appropriate treatment for your symptoms and a consistent bedtime are the best way to tackle sleep problems once and for all.

Strategies to help get a better night's sleep

Once you have looked at an effective treatment for your symptoms, attempted to establish a consistent sleeping

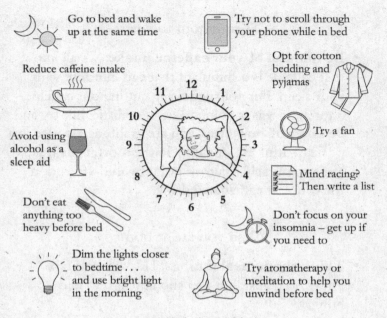

Go to bed and wake up at the same time

Try not to scroll through your phone while in bed

Reduce caffeine intake

Opt for cotton bedding and pyjamas

Try a fan

Avoid using alcohol as a sleep aid

Mind racing? Then write a list

Don't eat anything too heavy before bed

Don't focus on your insomnia – get up if you need to

Dim the lights closer to bedtime . . . and use bright light in the morning

Try aromatherapy or meditation to help you unwind before bed

Strategies for better sleep

pattern and tried to settle your racing mind, you should try some of the strategies given overleaf to maintain a good routine.

But this isn't about providing a list of things that you must do every single day before going to bed. While some repetition can be good, trying to change everything at once will only make you feel overwhelmed or anxious, which is the last thing you need when you are about to go to bed.

Read through the following suggestions, identify any tips that might work for you and take it from there.

Throughout the day

- **Be mindful of your caffeine intake**: We all know that caffeine is a stimulant that can interfere with your sleep. I'm not suggesting cutting out caffeine entirely, if this is going to be unrealistic, but try and be aware of how often you are grabbing a coffee, tea or fizzy-drink fix. A cuppa in the morning is fine, but set yourself a cut-off point by mid-afternoon for your last caffeinated drink.

When you are at home

- **Think about meal timings**: Heavy meals take longer to digest, but you shouldn't go to bed hungry.
- **. . . and go easy on the alcohol**: A few glasses of wine will initially make you drowsier and more relaxed, but alcohol disrupts the sleep cycle, leading to early waking and fatigue the following day.
- **Wind down and dim the lights**: Try using a dimmer switch in your living room and slowly dim the lights as bedtime approaches to help your body release the sleep chemical melatonin.

Creating the ideal sleep environment

- **Think about fabrics**: Choose cotton bedding and nightwear to keep the skin cool and to wick away sweat from the body. Some companies now make split-tog duvets, so that your partner can snuggle under a heavier tog while you keep cool lying under the more lightweight half, if that suits you better.

- **. . . and don't sleep naked**: Stripping off when you are feeling hot and bothered might sound appealing, but if you have night sweats, the sweat will remain on your skin and it will take longer to cool down.
- **Keep a fan close by**: Try having a fan on a low setting; it can help make your room cooler without the noise keeping you awake.

What to do if you wake up in the night

- **Have a change of scene**: There is no point lying in bed with your mind racing. Change your environment: get up and go to the bathroom, head to the kitchen and fix yourself a drink or read a book in the living room. When you feel sleepy again, go back to bed.
- **Don't forget about consistency**: As hard as it may be in the short term, try and keep to the same bedtime and wake-up time, even if you have been awake in the night.

<u>**Do you work shifts? Here's what**</u>
<u>**can work for you**</u>
Coping with sleep problems during the perimenopause is particularly tricky if you

work shifts. When I was a junior doctor on call at weekends I would start on Friday at 8 a.m. and wouldn't finish until 5 p.m. on the Monday. That feeling of battling against your own circadian rhythm and having to stay awake, when all I wanted to do was sleep, is something I will never forget.

If you are working night shifts, try introducing bright light in the evening before your shift starts, the Sleep Council advises.[6] And daylight suppresses melatonin production, so you can reduce exposure to the morning light on your way home from work by wearing sunglasses. When you get home, don't head straight to bed: allow yourself time to switch off and have something light to eat. If your family is working from home, ask them to try and keep the noise down, where possible, so they don't disturb your sleep time.

And follow a tip from the Health and Safety Executive:[7] don't be tempted to use your sleep time to catch up on jobs around the home. If necessary, change the times or days when some jobs are done.

8. Exercise for a Better Menopause

The perimenopause and menopause can send our motivation to exercise spiralling to an all-time low. After all, symptoms like fatigue, joint pain, hot flushes and vaginal dryness are hardly conducive to a vigorous workout. Even patients who are seasoned runners and cyclists say that their appetite for exercise wanes and, with it, their dreams of reaching their personal best.

But as you will see in this chapter, exercise can be an integral part of managing your perimenopause and menopause. Exercise boosts your physical and mental health and can help protect your body from the effects of hormone deficiency. After consulting a healthcare professional on the right treatment for you, you should hopefully see bothersome symptoms subside and your energy and appetite for activity should return. So whether you are a gym bunny or someone who hasn't exercised in a while, let's look at ways to build regular exercise into your life.

The benefits of exercise before and after the menopause

Exercise increases your heart rate and gets the blood flowing around your body. In response to any perceived stress or pain, the brain releases chemicals called endorphins. As well as acting as natural painkillers, endorphins have a positive effect on mood, giving you a high that helps you feel relaxed and more positive.

Exercise is also beneficial for bone health – a key concern, as women are more at risk of developing osteoporosis, where the bones lose their strength and break more easily in later life. As a living tissue, our bones strengthen when we use them. Regular exercise also lowers our risk of cardiovascular disease and dementia, as well as helping us maintain a healthy weight.

How much exercise should I aim for?

Current guidelines state that adults aged nineteen to sixty-four should be aiming for half an hour of moderate-intensity exercise five times a week, plus strength exercise at least two days a week.[1] Examples of moderate exercise include brisk walking, tennis, cycling and even mowing the lawn. Strength exercises include working with resistance bands, push-ups, sit-ups and lifting weights.

If you haven't exercised for a while, don't be daunted. Start small and build up to this level. Even adding a few minutes of running to the end of a daily walk is progress.

What exercises are important during perimenopause and menopause?

Unless you have been told by a healthcare professional to avoid a particular exercise, all exercise will be beneficial to your general health and well-being before, during and after your menopause.

In addition, there are two types of exercise that are particularly good for bone health. The first is weight-bearing exercise, where the bones support your weight. Examples of good weight-bearing exercise include brisk walking, dancing and aerobics. Variety is good for the bones, and you can achieve this by varying the movements, direction and speed.

The second type is strength exercise, where you use your muscles to pull on your bones. Your bones will respond to this by renewing themselves or by maintaining or improving their strength. Examples of strength activity include yoga, Pilates and exercises involving weights or resistance bands. The main thing is to find something you enjoy, so that you are more likely to stick with it – be that a dancing class or putting on a YouTube workout before the rest of the household wakes up.

Bone-strengthening exercises
Always remember to warm up and cool down before and after exercise to avoid injury.

1. Lie on your back with your hands at the sides, knees bent, hip-distance apart, and feet flat on the floor.

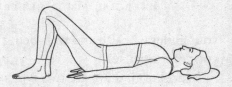

2. Tighten your tummy muscles and buttocks and lift your bottom up from the floor, towards the ceiling. Keep your shoulders on the floor and your knees close together, and aim for a straight line between your shoulders and knees, if this is comfortable.

3. Hold for up to 5 seconds, then gently lower back down to the floor.

4. Repeat up to 10 times.

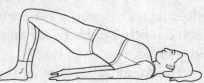

Bridge

1. Stand with your feet shoulder-width apart and with your arms out in front for balance.

2. Bend your knees as though you are going to sit on a chair and pause when your thighs are parallel to the floor. Keep your back straight and ensure that your knees don't extend over your toes.

3. Return to a standing position and repeat 10 times.

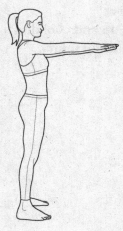

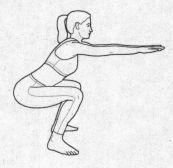

Squat

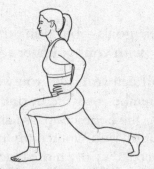

1. Looking straight ahead, take a step forward with one leg, lowering your hips until both knees are bent at about 90 degrees.

2. Be careful not to let your front knee lean over the toes as you lunge and keep your upper body upright at all times.

3. Change legs and repeat for a total of 10 times altogether.

Lunge

What should I be wearing?

You don't need to spend a fortune on a whole new workout wardrobe, but be mindful of what you wear when exercising, so that you don't exacerbate any symptoms and take the enjoyment out of the activity.

- If hot flushes are an issue, look for fabrics that will let the air circulate and any moisture evaporate, or simply opt for cotton.
- Protect your joints by wearing well-fitting, supportive shoes that won't put undue stress on your feet, ankles or knees.
- If vaginal dryness is a problem, avoid anything too tight-fitting.

Set yourself goals – but don't try to compete with your younger self

Maybe ten or fifteen years ago you were running marathons. But remember that the hormone deficiency that develops during the perimenopause and menopause can really take it out of you. Women often tell me how their stamina is reduced, they tire more quickly and their muscles and joints hurt for longer after exercise than they used to. If you have recently started taking HRT, then your symptoms will take a little while to subside, but the good news is that a lot of women who take HRT find that their exercise tolerance and stamina improve. Set yourself small goals until your energy returns and you can build up the level and frequency of your exercise.

- **Find the right time**: Schedule exercise into your day as you would a work meeting. That way it becomes part of your day, rather than an added extra to push further and further down your list of priorities until it drops off. Timing is also important: would fitting in twenty minutes in the morning be better than leaving exercise until later in the day? Could you do it in your lunch break?
- **It doesn't have to be all or nothing**: Try and build some movement into every day, whether it is walking or cycling where you can, taking the stairs or doing some stretches every few hours while you're working.

- **Build strength exercises into your daily life**: Try adding some strength exercises into other activities. I sometimes do simple exercises like squats, or even standing on one leg while drying my hair in the morning or waiting for the kettle to boil. Sure, I might get some odd looks from my husband and daughters, but it fills what would otherwise be dead time with repetitive movements that help keep my bones and muscles strong.

- **Give it a rest**: Just as we are at risk of burnout if we push ourselves too hard at work, the same can be said for our bodies. Having a day off to relax and recuperate is important to help our muscles recover.

Be kind to yourself

During the perimenopause and menopause we tend to be at an age when we are being pulled in so many different directions – by jobs, partners, children and relatives – that doing something just for ourselves seems impossible. But exercise is such an important investment in our health and well-being. Ensure you make some space for self-care and exercise, but be kind to yourself if life gets in the way of your exercise during a busy week.

Yoga

I have practised Ashtanga yoga for a long time and in recent years it has become a really important way to help manage my menopause and improve my health.

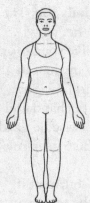

1. Stand tall with your feet together and your arms resting by your sides.

2. Fix your gaze on something in front of you and take some breaths, inhaling through the nose and exhaling through the mouth.

Slowly raise your right foot off the floor, positioning the sole on the inside of your left thigh.

The toes should be pointing down and your hips facing forward.

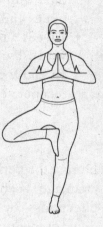

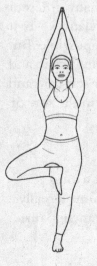

3. Inhale and raise your arms straight up towards the ceiling, with the palms pressed together. Hold for a few breaths.

Lower your arms and then slowly slide your right foot back down to the ground.

Repeat these steps with your left foot raised.

Tree pose

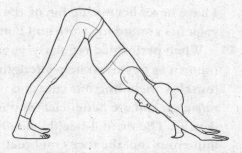

1. Starting on your hands and knees, tuck your toes under, and lift your hips up and back until your body forms a triangle. Use your core strength and your legs to bring the weight back as much as possible.

2. Stay for 5–8 breaths. With each breath try to press your heels towards the mat. Challenge yourself to push a little further each time but don't do anything that feels uncomfortable to your body. Lower down, and repeat twice more.

Downward dog

1. Start by kneeling on all fours.

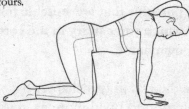

2. Slowly push your bottom back towards your heels. At the same time slide your hands in front of you, resting your forehead on the floor.

3. Hold this position for up to 30 seconds and then return to the starting position.

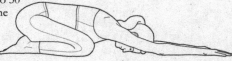

Child's pose

I have never been a big fan of the gym, and yoga fits around my work and home life.

When performed regularly, yoga movements (known as postures) help strengthen our muscles, including our core and pelvic-floor muscles, and are beneficial for our bone density. The mental-health benefits are numerous too: the focus on breathing helps to reduce anxiety and brings about a sense of calm. Women who attend the yoga sessions at my clinic say it also helps with sleep disturbance and hot flushes.

If you haven't tried yoga before, I would highly recommend trying out a class to see if it is something you enjoy. In the meantime, see the previous pages for three of my favourite postures that are suitable for beginners and which you can try in the comfort of your own home.

I hope the tips in this chapter have given you the tools and inspiration to build more exercise into your life. The physical and mental benefits are just too important to miss out on. Take exercise at your own pace, build it into your everyday routine and, above all, have fun!

9. Optimizing Your Nutrition during the Menopause

You can't predict when your menopause will happen or the symptoms you may experience. But the one thing you do have control over is your diet. Eating the right foods can help to strengthen your bones, improve the health of your cardiovascular system and regulate your mood.

Coupled with exercise (as discussed in the previous chapter), a well-balanced diet can help maintain a healthy weight and tackle the so-called middle-aged spread, when your metabolism often slows and your body responds to falling oestrogen levels by trying to build up a reserve of oestrogen in the fat cells. Whether you are in the middle of your menopause or preparing for the perimenopause, use this time to take stock of your overall diet.

I am not advocating embarking on a quick-fix diet, nor do I want you to count calories obsessively. Instead this chapter is all about looking at the vital nutrients and food choices that your body needs at this time, along with some simple changes you can make to stay nourished, strong and ready to cope with the menopause, as well as improve your future health.

Why it's time to rethink how you view food

So many of the women I see in my clinic find themselves caught up in an unhealthy cycle, when it comes to their diet. For some people, food and alcohol are a source of comfort or a form of reward after a hard day. For others, fatigue clouds their food choices and they opt for caffeine or sugar to give them a quick energy boost.

Spending hours cooking is probably the last thing you want to do when you feel tired, achy and are having yet another hot flush. Yet relying on processed and convenience foods that are high in sugar, salt and saturated fat will leave you feeling sluggish and unsatisfied. The sooner you start to see food as a form of medicine, the better. There is so much more to good menopause care than simply putting on a patch or taking a pill.

At my clinic we take a holistic approach to the menopause – and sound nutritional advice is a core part of that approach. That's because what we eat during the perimenopause and menopause directly impacts on the ways our body and mind deal with the challenges of the change, as well as impacting on our future health.

A good diet is all about balance and variety: think fresh fruits and vegetables packed with vitamins and nutrients, wholegrain foods that are high in fibre and give us energy, unsaturated fats and oils, and lean meat and fish.

Keep a food diary
Write down everything you eat and drink for a few days to assess how varied your diet is. Be honest and look for any gaps. Are you drinking enough water (about six to eight glasses a day)? Are you eating a variety of fruits and vegetables? Are your meals healthy, but a tendency to snack on processed foods lets you down?

The nutrients your body needs for a healthy, happy perimenopause and menopause

Below we look in more detail at the vital nutrients that can nourish and protect your body, at how much you should be aiming to eat and how you can build them into your everyday diet.

Calcium

Calcium helps build and maintain our bones – in fact 99 per cent of calcium in our body is stored in our bones. It is a hugely important mineral throughout our lives, but particularly during our menopause and post-menopause, when a lack of oestrogen leaves us at increased risk of osteoporosis.

- **How much do I need?** Guidelines state that women aged eighteen to sixty-four need about

700mg of calcium a day and should be able to get enough each day by eating a balanced diet.[1]
- **How do I get it?** Dairy products such as milk, cheese and yoghurt are well-known and important sources of calcium, but also leafy green vegetables, soya beans, nuts and fish.

Vitamin D

Vitamin D helps aids calcium absorption, so it supports strong bones. We get most of our vitamin D from exposure to sunlight – it is synthesized in the skin when it is exposed to sunlight that contains sufficient ultraviolet B (UVB) radiation, which usually occurs during the summer months.

- **How much do I need?** Guidelines state that everyone over the age of one should get about 10mcg (micrograms) of vitamin D a day.
- **How do I get it?** There are relatively few naturally rich sources of vitamin D in our food, although it can be found in egg yolk, meat, animal fat, liver, kidney and oily fish such as salmon and mackerel. Supplements are important because it is really difficult to obtain enough vitamin D from your diet, and it is also impossible to know how much vitamin D someone has made through their skin. In the UK it is recommended that everyone over the age of four takes a supplement between September and March.[2]

Magnesium

Magnesium is a mineral that is used throughout the body, including in our bones, brain and muscles. It converts the food we eat into energy and helps balance our blood glucose and regulate mood, promotes relaxation and aids sleep. Magnesium is also involved in building strong bones, as calcium and magnesium work together.

- **How much do I need?** Guidelines state that adult women aged nineteen to sixty-four need 270mg of magnesium a day.
- **How do I get it?** Magnesium is found in green leafy vegetables, nuts and seeds, squash, wholegrains, legumes and pulses. Bear in mind that alcohol, caffeinated drinks and medication such as antibiotics can affect magnesium absorption, as can stress. You might also consider taking a good-quality magnesium supplement – a lot of women that I talk to find it helps aid restful sleep and reduces the frequency of headaches and migraines.

Low-GI foods

The glycaemic index (GI) is a rating system for foods that contain carbohydrates, a key source of energy for the body. Foods with a high GI are digested more quickly and cause a rapid release of blood glucose, which can cause a sugar high or mood swings. Low-GI foods, on the other hand, are digested more slowly and release energy at a steadier rate, helping to stabilize blood glucose and mood.

- **What types of low-GI foods should I be eating?**
Try to avoid the white refined carbohydrates found in foods such as white bread, white rice and pizza. Switching to low-GI carbohydrates, such as wholegrain bread, brown rice, pulses, beans or sweet potatoes, will help maintain blood-sugar levels. You might also find that eating smaller meals more regularly helps to keep mood swings in check.

Fibre

Fibre is a type of carbohydrate. It is the part of fruits, vegetables and grains that cannot be digested by your stomach. Fibre helps to aid digestion, prevents constipation, helps us feel fuller and encourages the growth of good bacteria in the gut. It also has some important wider health benefits: it is associated with a lower risk of heart disease, stroke, Type 2 diabetes and bowel cancer.

- **How much do I need?** Current UK guidelines say that adults should be eating about 30g of dietary fibre a day as part of a healthy diet. To put that into context, two slices of wholemeal bread contain about 5g of fibre.
- **How do I get it?** Good sources of fibre include fruits and vegetables, wholegrains such as wholewheat pasta, bulgur wheat and brown rice, and legumes. *Tip*: If you are increasing the amount of

fibre in your diet, do it slowly but surely; suddenly introducing large amounts of fibre into your diet can cause bloating.

Omega-3

Omega-3 is a family of fatty acids found in foods and supplements. There are three main types: ALA (alpha-linolenic acid) cannot be made in the body, so it comes from our food alone; EPA (eicosapentaenoic acid) and DHA (docosahexaenoic acid) can be made from ALA in our bodies and are found in foods. Omega-3 has numerous benefits: it can help mood, circulation and is anti-inflammatory.

- **How much do I need?** Oily fish like mackerel and salmon are the prime source of EPA and DHA, and you should aim to eat at least one portion of oily fish a week.
- **How do I get it?** If you don't eat fish, ALA is found in vegetable oils, rapeseed and flaxseed, nuts such as walnuts, pecans and hazelnuts and in green leafy vegetables, or in supplements.

Phytoestrogens
Phytoestrogens are plant compounds that are similar in structure to the oestrogen that is naturally produced in our bodies, and to body-identical oestrogen. They are found in varying degrees in foods, including soy, legumes such as beans and lentils, and nuts and seeds.

When we eat phytoestrogens they are absorbed into the bloodstream and attach to oestrogen receptors throughout our bodies, producing an oestrogen-like effect. Ground flaxseeds sprinkled on your breakfast porridge or cereal, or used as a natural thickener to sauces, are a good way to add phytoestrogens to your diet.

Phytoestrogens are thought to help with hot flushes.[3] However, they are weaker than natural oestrogen or body-identical oestrogen.

Isoflavones – a type of phytoestrogen – are available as a supplement, but are not recommended for women with a history of breast cancer as there is no evidence to support its safety.

Be good to your gut

A common complaint that I hear in my clinic is of women suffering from persistent bloating, cramps, constipation or diarrhoea. Few women realize these symptoms can actually be related to their menopause.

We know how hormones play a part in everything from regulating our menstrual cycle to our mood. And our gastrointestinal system – the network involved in digesting and extracting vital nutrients and energy from food – is no exception. The part of our brain called the hypothalamus is involved in keeping our gastrointestinal system (commonly known as our gut) in check. The hypothalamus contains oestrogen receptors, so when oestrogen levels fluctuate during the menopause, this has a knock-on effect on gut function, resulting in sometimes painful symptoms.

How can I help my gut?

A poorly functioning gut won't absorb nutrients very well, so your stores of nutrients such as calcium and magnesium are at risk of becoming depleted.

1. **Correct your hormone deficiency:** Speak to a health professional about whether HRT is an option for you.
2. **Get some good bacteria:** Prebiotic foods, such as onions, garlic, asparagus, artichoke, chicory and banana, promote the growth of 'good' bacteria in your gut. Good bacteria can help boost immunity, energy and mood.

   Probiotic foods are fermented foods teeming with live bacteria and yeasts that help to balance bacteria in the gut. Examples of probiotic foods include live yoghurt, sauerkraut, kimchi and live apple-cider vinegar. If you have a sweet tooth you could try kombucha, a slightly fizzy fermented tea that makes a refreshing alternative if you are craving a fizzy drink or even a glass of wine.

Foods to limit

- **Ultra-processed foods**: Foods such as ready meals, cakes and pastries are high in sugar, salt and saturated fat and have little nutritional value. It is probably no surprise that studies show that regularly eating ultra-processed foods is linked to an increased risk of cardiovascular disease and weight gain. An occasional treat is fine, but if you regularly eat these foods, try taking your food diary a step further. How did you feel after eating the food? Did you reach for another snack soon afterwards?

- **Alcohol**: As we age, the body becomes more sensitive to alcohol because it holds less water to dilute it. Alcohol may help you unwind after a hectic day or moment, but it has a negative effect on your mood and mental health in the long run. Many menopausal women find that alcohol can be a trigger for, or increases the severity of, hot flushes and headaches. It can also interfere with sleep quality.

   There is a fine line between a 'moderate' amount of alcohol that is not associated with increased health risks and an excessive amount that has many potential risks. Remember that moderation is key: research shows that anything more than one small glass of wine per day (or one beer or single shot of spirit) can be identified as 'excessive'. Drinking more than this amount increases your risk of many types of cancer, heart disease, liver disease, osteoporosis, obesity and depression.

10. Going through the Menopause Due to Cancer Treatment

Being diagnosed with cancer can often be a time of huge upheaval, uncertainty and change. And one change that you may not have considered in those early days after your diagnosis is an early menopause.

If you have had a gynaecological cancer (uterine, ovarian, cervical, vaginal or vulval), then certain types of chemotherapy, radiotherapy or surgery may bring on symptoms of the menopause. There are also some types of drugs used in the treatment of breast cancer and other oestrogen receptor-positive cancers that block the action of certain hormones, often triggering menopausal symptoms while you are taking the treatment.

In sharp contrast to a natural menopause, which usually happens over a period of months and years, menopause due to medical treatment can happen quite suddenly. As Kelly, our case study on page 152 put it, 'For me it wasn't a menopause: it was a meno-stop.'

Symptoms such as hot flushes, vaginal dryness and mood changes can be distressing to cope with, alongside your cancer diagnosis and treatment. But the good news is that for most women there are very effective ways to help you cope with these symptoms while living with cancer, and to help safeguard your future health beyond cancer.

Why may cancer treatment affect when I go through the menopause?

Certain cancer treatments can stop the ovaries from working properly (either temporarily or permanently) and bring about an earlier menopause.

- **Surgery:** This includes an oophorectomy, where one or both ovaries are removed; you may also have one or both of your ovaries removed during a hysterectomy (when your uterus is removed). Having a hysterectomy and conserving your ovaries can also lead to an earlier menopause.
- **Types of chemotherapy:** As well as destroying cancer cells, chemotherapy can damage some healthy cells in the body. A woman's eggs are highly susceptible to the effects of certain types of chemotherapy, and this can result in the failure of the ovaries and an early menopause. The risk of this happening depends on the dose and duration of chemotherapy and on the type of chemotherapy being given. This is also more likely in women who already have a reduced reserve of eggs, such as older women.
- **Radiotherapy to the pelvic area:** Whereas most chemotherapy is administered throughout the body, radiotherapy tends to be directed at a particular area. Radiotherapy aimed at or around the ovaries can damage them enough to affect their function. High doses can destroy some or all of the eggs

in the ovaries, triggering menopausal symptoms. Even if the radiotherapy is not aimed directly at the ovaries, the rays can be absorbed and damage the ovaries.

- **Hormone treatments for breast cancer**: see the text below.

Hormone therapy

Some breast cancers are known as hormone receptor-positive cancers. Hormone treatments are often given to women who have had a hormone receptor-positive cancer. The way they work is more complicated than simply by blocking a hormone in the body, and different medications work in different ways. The type of hormone therapy you may have usually depends on:

- The stage and grade of the cancer
- Which hormone it is sensitive to
- Your age
- Whether you have experienced the meno-pause
- Other treatments that you are having.

Hormone therapy is usually given after surgery and chemotherapy, but in some cases it can be given before surgery to help shrink a tumour. Most women are advised to take hormone therapy for five years or more, after having surgery. Hormone therapies include:

- Tamoxifen: A hormone drug given to women who have had some types of breast and uterine cancer, taken daily as a tablet or liquid.
- Aromatase inhibitors: Tablets that block aromatase, a substance that helps the body to produce oestrogen after the menopause.
- Ovarian ablation or suppression: This stops the ovaries working and producing oestrogen. Ovarian ablation is done using surgery or radiotherapy and permanently stops the ovaries from working, triggering the menopause. Ovarian suppression usually involves a monthly injection of a medicine called goserelin. Your periods will stop while taking the medicine and should start again once treatment is complete. However, if you are approaching the age of the natural menopause (about fifty-one), then your periods may not start again.

Other frequently asked questions

Below are some questions that are commonly asked by women who are undergoing treatment for cancer.

How likely is it that I will go through an early menopause due to my treatment?

The likelihood depends on factors including your age, the type of treatment and your family history. In my clinic, and in my work raising awareness of the menopause, I have spoken to many women who have had cancer, from their teens up to their fifties, and there is no definitive answer. Just like the timing of the natural menopause, every woman's case is unique.

Will my menopause be temporary or permanent?

Again this depends on factors like your age and the type of treatment. If you have an oophorectomy or a hysterectomy where both ovaries are removed, then you will have your menopause immediately, regardless of your age. If one of your ovaries is left intact after an oophorectomy (or both are intact after a hysterectomy), there is a chance that you will experience the menopause within five years of having surgery.

The menopause after pelvic radiotherapy or chemotherapy could be temporary or permanent. This usually depends on how close you are to the age of your natural menopause and on the dose of radiation or the type of drugs used. Ovarian suppression can also be temporary or permanent, depending on how close you are to the age of your natural menopause.

If your menopause is temporary, then your periods may take several months, or even a few years, to return.

Will my fertility be affected?

Even if your fertility is not something you have thought or worried about, your specialist should be talking to you about how any treatment may affect your fertility.

I see women in my clinic who have, quite rightly, focused on their cancer and their treatment as their top priority. The whole issue of fertility has not been properly discussed, perhaps because they are quite young or they aren't with a partner at the time of their diagnosis, so the question of having children in the near future is not a consideration. And it may be that you do not want to have children in the near future, or even at all. But it is still crucial to have a conversation about your own individual circumstances, based on your age and treatment type.

Sadly, I have spoken to women whose circumstances change and because they haven't had this discussion, they then find it is too late, as their ovaries have been irreversibly damaged or removed.

What menopausal symptoms can I expect?

Your symptoms will mirror those of a natural menopause, although they may be more severe than for other women. Some of the most common symptoms for women with cancer include:

- Hot flushes
- Fatigue
- Joint pains and stiffness
- Night sweats
- Mood changes
- Period changes
- Vaginal dryness and other vaginal and urinary symptoms.

An early menopause can also put you at higher risk of long-term conditions such as osteoporosis and cardio-vascular disease.

How can I tell if my symptoms are due to the menopause or a side-effect of my treatment?

It can be hard to distinguish between treatment side-effects and menopausal symptoms. For example, an estimated nine in ten people suffer from cancer-related fatigue due to their treatment or the cancer itself.[1] Hot flushes, joint pain, brain fog, UTIs and vaginal dryness are all known side-effects of cancer treatment. Hot flushes are a common side-effect of chemotherapy, and vaginal dry-ness can be a particular problem for women who take the hormone-therapy drug tamoxifen (although this is usually directly related to the effects of this medication blocking oestrogen).

Then there is the psychological impact of your can-cer diagnosis and treatment. Younger women with an early menopause should also have a bone-density scan and FSH testing to help aid diagnosis. It's also import-ant that you talk to your healthcare professionals about any physical or mental-health concerns at the earliest opportunity.

If you can, record your symptoms using the menopause-symptom sheet on www.menopausedoctor.co.uk, or via my Balance app, ready to discuss it with your healthcare professional – having a fuller picture of the type, frequency and severity of your symptoms will help to plan a treatment approach.

How can I get help if I need it?

Menopause guidelines clearly state that women who are likely to go through the menopause as a result of medical or surgical treatment should be offered support. You should also be given information about the menopause before you have treatment, and should ideally be referred to a healthcare professional with expertise in menopause. You should expect to discuss:

- The risk of early menopause
- How your fertility might be affected
- Common menopausal symptoms
- Longer-term health implications of menopause
- Advice about contraception.

Sadly, this doesn't always happen for women. If you aren't getting the information and support you need, ask for a referral for specialist help.

> **<u>Forewarned is forearmed</u>**
> **Here are five key questions for your medical team:**
>
> 1. **Will my treatment trigger menopausal symptoms?**
> 2. **Will this be temporary or permanent?**

3. When will I be referred to a healthcare professional with expertise in menopause?
4. What treatment can I have if my menopausal symptoms affect my everyday life?
5. How will treatment affect my fertility [if applicable]?

Treatments

If you are menopausal due to your cancer treatment, please do not suffer in silence. Your symptoms may well be more severe than for other women, due to the sudden onset, and there are treatment options available to you. Talk to your medical team, keep a record of your symptoms and ask for specialist menopause help if you don't feel you are being heard.

HRT

HRT will help tackle most symptoms within a few weeks, although vaginal and urinary symptoms can take from three months up to a year to resolve. HRT will also help protect against osteoporosis and cardiovascular disease, which is especially important in women who go through an early menopause. If your cancer is not hormone-dependent, then you should be able to take HRT. Speak to a healthcare professional about your individual circumstances so that you can make an informed decision.

If you are taking HRT and feel that your symptoms aren't improving within a few months, speak to a healthcare professional. Going through your menopause at a younger age means that your body's requirement for hormones is usually greater, compared to older women. Potentially your HRT dose is too low – many young women actually need two or even three times more HRT than the average dose given to older women, because their hormone levels are lower at a younger age – so your dosage or delivery method may need adjusting.

If you have had a hormone-dependent cancer, you may still be able to take HRT, as there is no good-quality evidence showing that women have a worse outcome when they take HRT. Taking HRT needs to be an individualized decision between you and a menopause specialist. There are numerous benefits of taking HRT, and many women who are experiencing dreadful symptoms decide that taking HRT is worth the potential risks in order to feel better and see future health benefits.

Other treatments

There are some alternative prescription medications that can be taken for symptoms, if you are unable or choose not to take HRT.

Some women find their symptoms improve by stopping or changing the hormone treatment for their cancer. Often women are advised to stop taking their hormone treatment for around six weeks, to determine whether or not their menopausal symptoms are an effect of their hormone treatment. If you do this and feel better after this time, then talk to your doctor about stopping it altogether or taking an alternative hormone treatment. This includes some types of antidepressants, such as citalopram or venlafaxine, which can improve hot flushes, but may have side-effects such as nausea.

CBT (see page 102) is shown to help with the mood changes related to menopause, and a balanced diet and regular exercise are also key.

Testosterone

As well as regulating sex drive, testosterone also often helps with your mood, memory and concentration. Not all women will need testosterone, but talk to your healthcare professional if you are taking HRT and find that it alone is not helping with these symptoms. Testosterone is usually given as a cream or gel, or occasionally as an implant.

Treatments for vaginal dryness and urinary symptoms

Local oestrogen in the form of a cream, gel, vaginal tablet or ring inserted into the vagina can help to ease symptoms. Using oestrogen in this way is not the same as taking HRT, so it does not have the same associated risks. It can be safely used by the majority of women on a regular basis for a long period of time, which is important, as symptoms can continue when you are post-menopausal and often return when you stop treatment. Women who have had an oestrogen receptor-positive cancer in the past can still usually safely use vaginal oestrogens.

Another option for dryness symptoms are non-hormonal vaginal moisturizers and lubricants during sex. These products can be bought over the counter and can be used either alongside hormones or on their own (see Chapter 3 for more details on the different types and recommended brands).

Your symptoms should improve within a few weeks or months of treatment. See a healthcare professional if your symptoms do not get better, as they can be due to other conditions.

Kelly, 42

Kelly was thirty-eight when she was diagnosed with cervical cancer. The diagnosis was a shock: her son was only nine months old, it was early spring and she was busy planning her wedding that autumn. Kelly was given a 50/50 chance of the treatment being successful. She was also advised that she would be infertile after treatment and that time was of the essence, so there was no time to freeze any of her eggs. She focused her energies on staying positive and keeping as healthy as possible to help her body through the gruelling rounds of chemotherapy and radiotherapy.

Thankfully, the treatment was successful, and Kelly received the all-clear the month after her October wedding. At her first follow-up appointment, about a month after receiving the all-clear, her oncologist asked how she was feeling. Kelly had no cancer-type symptoms, but her joints ached – even her fingers – and she'd forget what she was saying midway through a sentence. 'I feel like I'm seventy years old,' she recalls saying.

Her oncologist replied that it was because, essentially, her body *was* now seventy years old. Because of her cancer treatment, Kelly's body was no longer producing sex hormones, and the lack of hormones was having an impact on everything from her joints to her memory. For Kelly, it wasn't a menopause; it was a sudden, sharp meno-stop. She hadn't gone through the menopause – she was immediately out the other side, with nothing left in the tank.

Her oncologist told her she needed to be on HRT – her health depended on it, and he would write to her GP. But even with that recommendation, Kelly's GP was seemingly scared and would only prescribe the lowest dose of HRT. Instead she was offered counselling and antidepressants. Kelly was already attending counselling privately and she refused the antidepressants, knowing from previous experience that they did not suit her.

After much reflection and research, Kelly realized she couldn't carry on living life as she was – she was trying to forge ahead in a new career and instead of making a positive impression, she was either on the verge of crying, ached all over, couldn't remember words or was so very tired all the time. She was still under forty years of age. She wasn't prepared to live like this any more, or put up with her GP saying that she should expect some side-effects from her treatment.

She really had to fight for a referral to an HRT specialist, and even then it was only after yet another letter from her oncologist that she was eventually referred to a specialist at her local hospital. Tests revealed that she was suffering from malabsorption of HRT, as her patches were not sticking on well. She tried alternative forms and dosages and, while there was some improvement in her symptoms, Kelly still felt she was not living the life she should. She felt overwhelmed by all the information available online and almost gave up, but then made an appointment at my clinic.

We altered Kelly's HRT, by increasing her oestrogen dose and adding testosterone, and her symptoms have now subsided. She feels as if she has her life back: she has excelled professionally and has dealt with some very stressful work challenges that simply would not have been possible before.

Kelly is passionate that women going through the menopause should receive expert advice from the very start. Her advice to women in the same position? If you feel you aren't being listened to, then ask for a second opinion and push for a specialist referral. Do your research, and remember that *you* are the best expert in knowing how you feel.

11. Questions to Ask Your Healthcare Professional

If you are struggling with symptoms, then making an appointment with a healthcare professional should be an important turning point in your perimenopause or menopause journey. It should be where you receive a diagnosis and talk through the right treatment for you, to ease your symptoms and safeguard your future health.

Sadly, not all women have a positive experience. A 2020 survey of 1,500 women in the UK by Mumsnet and Gransnet found that many women are struggling to get appropriate help from GPs for perimenopausal and menopausal symptoms.[1] One-third of those sought help from their GP for perimenopause symptoms; and 26 per cent of those who sought help for menopause symptoms said they visited their GP three times or more before being prescribed appropriate medication or help.

There are many healthcare professionals dedicated to providing the best possible care for women. However, a huge knowledge gap exists around the perimenopause and menopause, not just in society in general, but also in the lack of formal menopause training for many healthcare professionals.

Overcoming a lack of expertise

Traditionally menopause care has been led by gynaecologists. I know that my menopause training at medical school, and while I worked in both hospital medicine and general practice, was non-existent. This means that women often don't get the right diagnosis and the correct treatment. I frequently see women who have consulted numerous other specialists and have undergone (often expensive) investigations, such as brain scans for migraines, heart scans for palpitations, bladder scans for urinary incontinence and needless blood tests.

One of my patients sought help more than a dozen times in two years with menopause-related memory problems. By the time she came to see me she had convinced herself she had dementia, as her memory was so dreadful. The menopause had never been mentioned, and she didn't think to tell healthcare professionals about her hot flushes, as she didn't know the two symptoms could be linked. None of the doctors she visited ever asked her about her periods.

Another issue is that many doctors are not referring to the most up-to-date evidence on menopause treatments, including HRT. There remains a reluctance to prescribe HRT, based on the misreported findings of studies and poor-quality research about HRT risks. This despite the fact that the current menopause guidelines state that, for the majority of women, the benefits of HRT outweigh any risks.

There is a danger that women are put off from seeking help, and this is having disastrous implications for their current and future health. As one woman who responded to the Mumsnet/Gransnet survey put it: 'I feel like I'm going insane, but do not feel that it's even worth another GP visit to try to sort it out.' I'm passionate that no woman should ever have to feel like this.

In addition to better menopause education for health-care professionals, I believe that, as women, we need to take steps to ensure we have a fruitful doctor's appointment and get access to the help we both need and deserve. After reading this book you should be empowered with knowledge about the perimenopause and menopause: you will know the common symptoms, the various treatments and their benefits and risks, based on your own circumstances. Above all, you know your own body and should ask yourself – and your healthcare professional – the key question: Could my symptoms be the perimenopause or menopause?

In this chapter we will look at your all-important doctor's appointment: how you can prepare, what you can expect to discuss, a checklist of key questions to ask and how to make sure you get the best treatment for you.

Where do I turn for help?

If you are based in the UK your first port of call will usually be your local GP practice, where your care will generally be overseen by a doctor or nurse. If you live elsewhere in the world, check in with your medical team to discuss who is the most appropriate person to see. At your initial appointment you and your healthcare professional should go over your symptoms and discuss any treatments or support, so that you can decide together what is best for you.

You should also expect to discuss at this appointment, or be given information to take home with you, details about:

- Menopause stages, symptoms and diagnosis
- Benefits and risks of different treatments, including HRT, non-hormone treatments and CBT
- Lifestyle changes that could help you
- The impact of the menopause on your long-term health.[2]

What happens next?

You should get booked in for a review three months after the initial appointment in which you are given treatment. This can then move to an annual review, if you are happy with your symptoms and the treatment you have been given. However, I would urge you to book an appointment sooner if you are worried about any side-effects from treatment or new symptoms – and always make sure you attend any regular screening appointments for your general health, such as a cervical smear test or breast-cancer screening.

When you might need a specialist referral

There are some cases when you may need to be referred to a menopause specialist. This can include if you have early menopause or suspected POI, or if your symptoms have been triggered by cancer or surgery. You can also be referred later down the line, if any treatments don't seem to be helping.

In the UK this will probably be a menopause clinic that includes healthcare professionals who specialize in more complex menopause cases, such as POI. You cannot self-refer to an NHS specialist menopause clinic; only a healthcare professional can do this. Another option is a private menopause clinic like mine, to which you can self-refer. The British Menopause Society website (see page 179) has a list of menopause clinics.

If you live elsewhere in the world, speak to your medical team if you believe that you need to see a menopause specialist.

Six steps to a successful first appointment

Work through the following steps to get the most out of the initial appointment with your healthcare specialist.

Step 1: Ask to see the most appropriate person

When you call to make your appointment, ask who is the most appropriate person to talk through your symptoms with and receive treatment from. You may find there is a doctor or nurse with a special interest in menopause.

Step 2: Lots to talk about? Request a double appointment

You will probably have to wait longer for a double appointment, but it could be worth it in the long run. Feeling that you are not up against the clock can help you relax. Your healthcare professional will probably be grateful too – I know, from my time as a GP, that one ten-minute appointment simply wasn't enough time to go through the symptoms of many women, let alone take a detailed health history and then discuss potential treatments. Alternatively, you may need to book two separate appointments.

Step 3: Prepare

Medical appointments are usually brief – often lasting just ten minutes. With such limited time it is easy to get flustered and feel as if you aren't being listened to. That is why preparation is key. Write down a list of your most troublesome symptoms – using the symptoms sheet on pages 13–15 of this book, by downloading it from my website (www.menopausedoctor.co.uk) or by using the free Balance app (balance-app.com) – and bring it with you to your appointment. You can also download and print off your Health Report from the Balance app, which will be really useful for this appointment.

Before your appointment (ideally the day before) take some time to read through your list. What symptoms are causing you the most discomfort or concern? Put them at the top of your list or highlight them, so that you focus on them first.

Remember that, for the majority of women, your diagnosis will be made on account of your age and symptoms. Having a comprehensive list will help your healthcare professional reach the right diagnosis and you can then spend more time discussing treatment options.

Step 4: Be open and honest about all your symptoms

I know that talking about your plummeting sex drive, vaginal dryness or mood swings can be daunting, but it is so important to be honest about all your symptoms, so that you can move on to the best treatment for you. Please don't feel embarrassed. Healthcare professionals are highly trained, very experienced and are there to help. Take a deep breath and go for it!

Step 5: Take notes – and ask questions

Make sure you fully understand the outcome of your appointment before you leave the room. As healthcare professionals, we know that the more understanding a patient has about their diagnosis and treatment, the better. Ask if there are any leaflets you can take away, or jot down some notes in a notepad or on your phone. This is particularly helpful if you are suffering from brain fog.

Step 6: Not satisfied with the outcome or advice? Ask for a second opinion

If your appointment has gone well – fantastic! But if it hasn't gone quite as you imagined, don't be afraid to challenge conclusions or treatment decisions. It is important that it is a two-way discussion.

HRT is not always going to be suitable for everyone as a first-line treatment, but if you feel you would benefit from taking HRT and your doctor or other healthcare professional refuses to prescribe it, ask if that decision is being made in line with current menopause guidelines. Likewise, if antidepressants are being offered, double-check the rationale behind this. If it is for menopause-related low mood, then this is not recommended. Do be mindful that there are reasons why antidepressants may be prescribed, such as to manage hot flushes in women who are unable to take HRT or for clinical depression.

You can always ask for a second opinion, either by seeing someone else at the same surgery or by requesting a referral to a specialist menopause clinic. Another option is self-referring to a private menopause clinic.

Marie, 51

Marie is a marketing director and had always enjoyed good health. About five years ago she started to experience a number of symptoms that she now knows were due to the perimenopause: a tightness in her chest, painful joints, pins and needles in her fingers and toes, and a burning sensation in the palms of her hands and soles of her feet. She was also experiencing a sensation of things crawling over her skin. The symptoms would come and go, but recently they had increased in frequency.

Marie made an appointment to see her doctor. He immediately diagnosed her symptoms as stress-related, and she left with an inhaler for the tightness in her chest and the offer of antidepressants, which she declined. She says she felt deflated and that the appointment had been a waste of time. Her symptoms continued, and different ones began to emerge. She was becoming forgetful, wasn't sleeping well and suffered from hot flushes.

At this point, about a year on from her initial appointment, Marie made an appointment with a different doctor at her surgery. This time the doctor was more sympathetic. Some twenty years earlier Marie had been referred to a neurologist because of inflammation in her optic nerve, which can be a sign of multiple sclerosis (MS). Fortunately, MS was ruled out and Marie returned to full health. Because of her history, and her current symptoms, the doctor again referred her to a neurologist. The neurologist couldn't find a root cause and Marie's doctor suggested that she would benefit from antidepressants. Again Marie refused these, because she truly did not believe she was depressed.

Not long afterwards she happened to catch a TV programme about the menopause and described it as a light-bulb moment; she recognized her symptoms as the perimenopause because she was still having periods. She changed her diet, tried to exercise more and took supplements. Nothing seemed to help. Marie was on the verge of quitting her job, avoided family and friends, and said she felt as if all the joy had been sucked out of her life.

By chance she was due to have a private annual 'well woman' check as part of her job. She broke down and told the doctor how awful she felt. The doctor confirmed that she was perimenopausal and said it would be beneficial for Marie to speak to someone about the possibility of HRT. Her healthcare package didn't cover menopause care, so she would have to go to an NHS doctor or pay for private care. Marie called her surgery as soon as she got home, but was told that the surgery did not support the prescribing of HRT.

At this point she contacted my clinic for an appointment. I prescribed oestrogen gel and a micronized progesterone tablet, and Marie was given a detailed letter to take to her GP so that her medical file was up to date. Sadly, when she made an appointment with her GP, she was again told that her symptoms were probably due to anxiety or depression. Her GP spoke about the risks of HRT, and that she would only support a prescription for it after Marie had tried antidepressants.

This was incorrect advice, so Marie saw another doctor in the same practice, who agreed that HRT would be the best treatment for her. She has continued with this and feels so much better. She is pleased that she persevered with finding another doctor who listened and understood.

Ten key questions to ask your doctor, to get advice and treatment tailored to you

There is no such thing as one-size-fits-all when it comes to good menopause care, and it is vital that women are involved from the outset in decisions about their care.

NICE's menopause guidelines apply specifically to the UK, but they include some really useful key questions that you can ask your healthcare professional at your first appointment, regardless of where you live.[3] Here are ten questions worth asking to ensure that you are receiving appropriate, individualized care.

1. How are you diagnosing my perimenopause or menopause?
2. Can you reach a diagnosis if I am taking a hormone treatment (such as the contraceptive pill)?

3. What types of treatment are suitable for my symptoms?
4. What are the benefits and risks of different treatments?
5. Can you tell me why you are/aren't recommending hormone HRT?
6. If I don't want to take HRT, or can't for medical reasons, what other treatments are there?
7. How quickly can I expect my symptoms to improve?
8. Are there any long-term effects of taking HRT?
9. Are there any support organizations in my local area?
10. Would you recommend any lifestyle changes to help my menopausal symptoms?

Conclusion

Whether you are in the early days of your perimenopause or reaching the end of your menopause, I hope the information and advice in this book have given you the clarity and confidence to take charge of your own health.

The women whose stories I have shared all faced setbacks and struggles in securing a diagnosis and the right treatment. Thankfully they found support, relief from their symptoms and the right treatment for them, resulting in their lives being transformed. I witness such transformations every day in my clinic. Women who had been on the verge of quitting their jobs, or ending relationships, regain their confidence and zest for life within a few months.

With the right treatments and a holistic approach to our health and well-being, the menopause doesn't have to be something to be endured – it really can be an enjoyable time of your life. Below are my four takeaways for a healthy, happy menopause.

- **Don't delay in seeking help and advice:**
  The days of struggling on in silence must be put behind us. No matter your age or your symptoms, if it is affecting your everyday life, please see a healthcare professional. Never wait until your symptoms become unbearable.

- **You are the expert when it comes to your mind and body:** If you 'don't feel quite right', speak up. Use the tools at your disposal – the menopause symptom sheet on the www.menopausedoctor.co.uk website, the symptom record on the Balance app or just an old-fashioned pen and paper. Record the type and severity of your symptoms. Take your list to any appointments and refer back to it, even after treatment starts, to make sure you are getting the best possible results.
- **Remember that good menopausal care isn't just about medicine:** Use this period in your life to reflect on your overall health and well-being. HRT remains the gold-standard treatment for hormone deficiency, but a good diet and regular exercise are essential for all women, regardless of whether or not they take HRT. Not only will they help you feel better in the short term, but a good diet and regular exercise can help protect against long-term health risks such as osteo-porosis and cardiovascular disease. And don't neglect your mental health. Book in regular time-out to do things you enjoy, to boost your self-esteem.
- **Talk about your experiences with others:** Slowly but surely, society is getting better at talking openly about the menopause. Well-known figures – including the TV presenters Lorraine Kelly and Davina McCall and the wellness expert Liz Earle – have all spoken candidly about their own menopause experiences. Thanks to campaigners, the menopause will be taught in secondary-school sex-and-relationship lessons in the UK, which is a huge

step forward. But we can all play a part in raising awareness – be it in the workplace, among friends or around the dinner table.

Looking ahead to your post-menopausal years

The post-menopause is defined as the time after you have not had a period for twelve consecutive months. Studies show that about 80 per cent of women will be post-menopausal by the age of fifty-four.[1] This of course can vary, so keep track of your menopause symptoms. You might find that symptoms subside over time and your energy levels and libido return.

However, issues such as vaginal dryness may persist long-term, so it is important to continue any treatments. Both hormone and non-hormone treatments are available – revisit Chapter 3 on 'taboo' symptoms for a refresher.

Remember: you can take HRT long-term
You can continue to take HRT for as long as the benefits outweigh the risks. If you do continue to take HRT or any other treatment, make sure you attend an annual review. And remember that if you have experienced an early menopause or have POI, it is recommended that you take hormones until at least the age of fifty-one, the natural age of the menopause.

Notes

1. Change before 'The Change': the Perimenopause

1 Faculty of Sexual and Reproductive Healthcare (2017, amended 2019), 'FSRH Clinical Guideline: Contraception for women aged over 40 years', www.fsrh.org/standards-and-guidance/documents/fsrh-guidance-contraception-for-women-aged-over-40-years-2017
2 Office for National Statistics (2019), 'Birth characteristics in England and Wales: 2017', www.ons.gov.uk/peoplepopula tionandcommunity/birthsdeathsandmarriages/livebirths/bulletins/birthcharacteristicsinenglandandwales/2017#:~:text=The%20average%20age%20of%20first,or%20subsequent%20births%20in%202017
3 Family Planning Association/FPA (2015), 'Your guide to male and female sterilisation', www.fpa.org.uk/sites/default/files/male-and-female-sterilisation-your-guide.pdf

2. What to Expect: Common Symptoms You Need to Know About

1 Women's Health Concern (2015), 'The Menopause', www.womens-health-concern.org/help-and-advice/factsheets/menopause
2 World Health Organization and Lifting the Burden (2011), 'Atlas of headache disorder and resources in the world

2011', www.who.int/mental_health/management/who_atlas_headache_disorders.pdf?ua=1

3 S. R. Davis, C. Castelo-Branco, P. Chedraui et al. (2012), 'Understanding weight gain at menopause', *Climacteric*, 15 (5), pp.419–29

4 Z. Hodson and L. Beveridge (2020), *Newson Health: Changing body shape during menopause* (booklet), www.menopausedoctor. co.uk/media/files/Booklets-with-copyright/Changing-Body-Shape-During-the-Menopause.pdf

5 U. Seeland, F. Coluzzi, M. Simmaco, C. Mura, P. E. Bourne et al. (2020), 'Evidence for treatment with estradiol for women with SARS-CoV-2 infection', *BMC Medicine*, doi: 10.1186/s12916-020-01851-z

6 National Institute for Health and Care Excellence (NICE) (2020), 'COVID-19 rapid guideline: Managing the long-term effects of COVID-19', www.nice.org.uk/guidance/NG188

7 N. Nabavi, 'Long covid: How to define it and how to manage it' (2020), *British Medical Journal*, www.bmj.com/content/370/bmj.m3489; C. H. Sudre, B. Murray, T. Varsavsky, M. S. Graham, R. S. Penfold, R. C. Bowyer et al. (2020), 'Attributes and predictors of Long-COVID: Analysis of COVID cases and their symptoms collected by the Covid Symptoms Study App', doi.org/10.1101/2020.10.19.20214494

3. Spotlight on Taboo Symptoms

1 North American Menopause Society (2020), 'How Important Is Sex to Women as They Age?', www.menopause.org/

docs/default-source/press-release/sex-importance-to-women-during-midlife-9-22-20.pdf

4. HRT and Other Treatment Options to Consider

1 NICE (2015), *Menopause: Diagnosis and management*, NICE guideline NG23, www.nice.org.uk/guidance/NG23

2 G. P. Cumming, H. Currie, E. Morris et al. (2015), 'The need to do better – are we still letting our patients down and at what cost?', *Post Reproductive Health*, 21 (2), pp.56–62

3 British Menopause Society (2019), 'Bioidentical HRT', BMS consensus statement, thebms.org.uk/publications/consensus-statements/bioidentical-hrt/

4 L. Newson and J. Rymer (2019), 'The dangers of compounded bioidentical hormone therapy', *British Journal of General Practice*, 69 (888), pp.540–41

5 NICE (2015), *Menopause: Diagnosis and management*

6 K. Maclaran and J. C. Stevenson (2012), 'Primary prevention of cardiovascular disease with HRT', *Women's Health*, 8, pp.63–74

7 NICE (2015), *Menopause: Diagnosis and management*

8 Women's Health Initiative (2019), 'Hormone therapy trials', www.whi.org/about/SitePages/HT.aspx

9 Collaborative Group on Hormonal Factors in Breast Cancer (2019), 'Type and timing of menopausal hormone therapy and breast cancer risk: Individual participant meta-analysis of the worldwide epidemiological evidence', *The Lancet*, 394 (10204), pp.1159–68

10 R. T. Chlebowski, G. L. Anderson, A. K. Aragaki et al. (2020), 'Association of Menopausal Hormone Therapy with Breast Cancer Incidence and Mortality During Long-term Follow-up of the Women's Health Initiative Randomized Clinical Trials', *Journal of the American Medical Association*, 324(4), pp. 369–80, doi:10.1001/jama.2020.9482

11 NICE (2015), *Menopause: Diagnosis and management*

12 Ibid.

13 Ibid.

5. Advice for Women Going through an Early Menopause

1 Daisy Network, 'What is POI?', www.daisynetwork.org/about-poi/what-is-poi

2 J. C. Gallagher (2007), 'Effect of early menopause on bone mineral density and fractures', *Menopause*, 14 (3 Pt 2), pp. 567–71

3 D. Zhu et al. (2019), 'Age at natural menopause and risk of incident cardiovascular disease: A pooled analysis of individual patient data', *The Lancet Public Health*, 4, pp. 553–64

4 NICE (2015), *Menopause: Diagnosis and management*, www.nice.org.uk/guidance/NG23

6. Menopause and Mental Health

1 Office for National Statistics (2019), 'Suicides in England and Wales: 2019 registrations', www.ons.gov.uk/people populationandcommunity/birthsdeathsandmarriages/

deaths/bulletins/suicidesintheunitedkingdom/2019 registrations

2 M. Leonhardt (2019), 'Low mood and depressive symptoms during perimenopause – should general practitioners prescribe hormone replacement therapy or antidepressants as the first-line treatment?', *Post Reproductive Health*, 25 (3), pp. 124–30

3 NICE (2015), *Menopause: Diagnosis and management*, www.nice.org.uk/guidance/NG23

4 Ibid.

5 C. M. van Driel, A. Stuursma, M. J. Schrovers et al. (2019), 'Mindfulness, cognitive behavioural and behaviour-based therapy for natural and treatment-induced menopausal symptoms: A systematic review and meta-analysis', *BJOG*, 126, pp.330–39

6 R. Sood, C. L. Kuhle, E. Kapoor, J. M. Thielen, K. S. Frohmader, K. C. Mara, S. S. Faubion (2019), 'Association of mindfulness and stress with menopausal symptoms in midlife women', *Climacteric*, 22 (4), pp.377–82

7. Menopause and Sleep

1 F. C. Baker, M. de Zambotti, I. M. Colrain et al. (2018), 'Sleep problems during the menopausal transition: Prevalence, impact, and management challenges', *Nature and Science of Sleep*, 10, pp.73–95

2 NICE (2020), 'Insomnia: Summary', cks.nice.org.uk/topics/insomnia/#!backgroundSub

3 M. Ohayon, E. Wickwire, M. Hirshkowitz et al. (2017), 'National Sleep Foundation's sleep quality recommendations: First report', *Sleep Health*, 3 (1), pp.6–19

4 P. Polo-Kantola, R. Erkkola, K. Irjala, S. Pullinen, I. Virtanen, O. Polo (1999), 'Effect of short-term transdermal estrogen replacement therapy on sleep: A randomized, double-blind crossover trial in postmenopausal women', *Fertility and Sterility*, 171, pp.873–80

5 Christopher M. Depner et al. (2019), 'Ad libitum weekend recovery sleep fails to prevent metabolic dysregulation during a repeating pattern of insufficient sleep and weekend recovery sleep', *Current Biology*, 29 (6), pp.957–67

6 The Sleep Council, 'Sleep Advice for Shift Workers', sleepcouncil.org.uk/advice-support/sleep-advice/common-sleep-scenarios/sleep-advice-for-shift-workers/

7 Health and Safety Executive, 'Hints and tips for shiftworkers', www.hse.gov.uk/humanfactors/topics/shiftworkers.htm

8. Exercise for a Better Menopause

1 NHS (2018), 'Physical activity guides for adults', www.nhs.uk/live-well/exercise

9. Optimizing Your Nutrition during the Menopause

1 Public Health England (2016), 'Government recommendations for energy and nutrients for males and females aged

1–18 years and 19+ years', assets.publishing.service.gov.uk/government/uploads/system/uploads/attachment_data/file/618167/government_dietary_recommendations.pdf

2 Scientific Advisory Committee on Nutrition (2016), 'Vitamin D and Health', assets.publishing.service.gov.uk/government/uploads/system/uploads/attachment_data/file/537616/SACN_Vitamin_D_and_Health_report.pdf

3 M. N. Chen, C. C. Lin, C. F. Liu (2015), 'Efficacy of phytoestrogens for menopausal symptoms: A meta-analysis and systematic review', *Climacteric*, 18 (2), pp.260–69

10. Going through the Menopause Due to Cancer Treatment

1 Macmillan Cancer Support (2018), 'Tiredness (fatigue)', www.macmillan.org.uk/cancer-information-and-support/impacts-of-cancer/tiredness

11. Questions to Ask Your Healthcare Professional

1 Mumsnet (2020), 'Women are struggling to get appropriate help from GPs for perimenopause and menopause symptoms', www.mumsnet.com/campaigns/gps-and-menopause-survey

2 NICE (2015), *Menopause: Diagnosis and management*, www.nice.org.uk/guidance/NG23

3 NICE (2015), 'Questions to ask about the menopause', in *Menopause: Diagnosis and management, information for the public*, www.nice.org.uk/guidance/ng23/ifp/chapter/questions-to-ask-about-menopause

Further Reading and Resources

General information on perimenopause and menopause

My Menopause Doctor, www.menopausedoctor.co.uk
The Menopause Charity, www.themenopausecharity.org
Balance app, www.balance-app.com
British Menopause Society, thebms.org.uk
International Menopause Society, www.imsociety.org
Menopause Support, www.menopausesupport.co.uk
North American Menopause Society, www.menopause.org
Canadian Menopause Society, www.sigmamenopause.com

Menopause guidelines

National Institute for Health and Care Excellence (NICE),
    www.nice.org.uk/guidance/ng23. *Menopause: Diagnosis and
    management*
NICE, www.nice.org.uk/guidance/ng23/ifp/chapter/
    Premature-menopause-premature-ovarian-insufficiency. *Pre-
    mature menopause (premature ovarian insufficiency)*
IMS recommendations on women's midlife health and meno-
    pause hormone therapy: https://www.imsociety.org/
    manage/images/pdf/4429e3dd302aac259ad68c3be7f60599.
    pdf

Menopause for younger women

Daisy Network, www.daisynetwork.org. A charity for women
with POI

Teenage Cancer Trust, www.teenagecancertrust.org. Special-
ized nursing care and support for teenagers

Trekstock, www.trekstock.com. Young adult cancer support

Health and well-being resources

Royal Osteoporosis Society, theros.org.uk/information-and-
support/bone-health/exercise-for-bones. Exercise that's
good for your bones

Emma Ellice-Flint nutrition, www.emmasnutrition.com. Food
secrets for a balanced life

Dinah Simon, @menopausepilates. Instagram account of
yoga and Pilates teacher, and founder of Menopause Pilates,
Dinah Simon

Dr Sally Norton, www.drsallynorton.com. Website of Dr Sally
Norton, consultant surgeon and weight-loss expert

Living Your Yoga, www.livingyouryoga.co.uk. Yoga resources
and classes from yoga teacher Lucy Holtom

Menopause Yoga, www.menopause-yoga.com. Website of yoga
teacher Petra Coveney

Yoga by Claudia, www.yogabyclaudia.com. Website of yoga
teacher Claudia Brown

Liz Earle Wellbeing, www.lizearlewellbeing.com. Food, beauty
and healthy-living content from researcher, writer and broad-
caster, Liz Earle

Acknowledgements

My mission to improve the global health of women is no mean feat, but I am a determined person and will not easily be beaten. However, I would achieve nothing without the tremendous help and guidance of so many people. Over the past few years there have been many occasions when I have received negative and hostile comments from the media, from work colleagues and also from women. These comments have often doubted my ability and my ambition.

The first person I would like to thank is my long-suffering husband, Paul. Over the past thirty-two years he has given me unlimited encouragement and support in all my work. He continues to listen endlessly to my frustrations, and persuades me to continue at times when I have actually felt like giving up my work.

My three children, Jess, Sophie and Lucy, have always listened to me talk tirelessly about the menopause, and they all continue to encourage me so much with my work, for which I am very grateful. My mother has always been there to ensure that I do my best and she is also one of the world's greatest advocates of HRT – she has spoken about this on one of my podcasts and also features as three different 'patients' on the menopause education programme we have developed! Sarah, John and Kay have all helped encourage me to persist and continue with my work. I am hoping that my father, who died when I was young, would be proud of this book, and I thank him for still being there to guide me.

I am extremely grateful to Dr Rebecca Lewis for being such an advocate as well as a close friend. She is often the voice of reason and gives me so much inner strength and confidence. Other doctors have helped me, both by creating the menopause education programme for healthcare professionals and by giving me advice, including Sarah Ball and Alice Duffy, as well as the other doctors and clinicians working with me in my menopause clinic.

I am appreciative of the mentoring that I receive from the USA from Avrum Bluming, Philip Sarrel and James Simon, who have so much knowledge and experience that they constantly share with me.

I would also like to thank Jane and Chris Oglesby, who have given me so much time, guidance and encouragement as well as so generously funding the development of the Balance app.

Much of my media work has been supported by the most inspirational women, including Liz Earle, Lorraine Kelly, Davina McCall and Kate Muir, and I am very appreciative of all their encouragement.

One of my greatest mentors is Professor Matthew Cripps, who is untiring in his belief in my work and has taught me so much about how to change people who do not want to be changed. This book will hopefully help some of those people!

I would also like to acknowledge Stacy Tuohy, Jackie Quinn, Kate Parr, Linda Daly, Abigail Moran, Sarah Kent, Lucy Chatwin, Gaele Lalahy, Katrina Palmer, Sarah Baker,

ACKNOWLEDGEMENTS

Alice Sievier, Lauren Lunn Farrow, Andrew Humphries, James Critchlow, Marcus Daly, Laura Harper, Zoe Hodson, Jane and Chris Oglesby and Vanessa Barnes, who know me in different ways, but I would be lost without them all.

However, none of my work would be possible without all my patients and the women who connect with me on social media, who I learn from every day. I would like to thank them all for providing me with the determination to keep working hard to increase their knowledge and reduce suffering in the future.

Finally, I would like to publicly thank Kat Keogh, who is the contributing editor of this book and whose knowledge, patience and professionalism have been outstanding and exceptional. My thanks also go to the team at Penguin who have made the experience of writing this book so enjoyable and rewarding.

MANAGING YOUR MIGRAINE
DR KATY MUNRO

Part of the Penguin Life Experts series.

Despite being one of the most common and debilitating conditions in the world, migraine is still widely misunderstood, stigmatized and misdiagnosed. Migraine is much more than 'just a headache', so why do we still know so little about this genetic neurological brain disorder and its causes? Headache specialist and GP Dr Katy Munro has the answers you're looking for.

Managing Your Migraine is the practical go-to guide for understanding migraine, equipping readers with practical, expert advice.

If you're a person with migraine, or know someone struggling, this book will provide helpful strategies for alleviating and managing your symptoms. Drawing on her medical expertise, her own personal experience with migraine and the stories of her patients, Dr Munro will empower you to get to know your own migraine and build an effective treatment plan that will help you to live your life to the full.